Homeopathic Medicine Chest

Ambika Wauters, R. S. Hom.

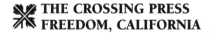

THE CROSSING PRESS
FREEDOM, CALIFORNIA

For information on bulk purchases or group discounts for this and other Crossing Press titles, please contact our Special Sales Manager at 800-777-1048.

Visit our Website on the Internet at: **www.crossingpress.com**

Library of Congress Cataloging-in-Publication Data

Wauters, Ambika.
    Homeopathic first aid / by Ambika Wauters.
        p. cm.
    ISBN 1-58091-055-6 (pbk.)
      1. Homeopathy. 2. Homeopathy—Materia medica and therapeutics.
3. First aid in illness and injury. I. Title.

RX71.W38   2000
615.5'32—dc21   99-054239
                                                            CIP

Contents

What Is Homeopathy?

Homeopathy is a complete medicine which, when used intelligently, will heal many conditions. It can be used by anyone of any age to restore balance and well-being. It is a medicine that is both life-enhancing and revitalizing, bringing harmony to stressed bodies, frazzled nerves, and weary spirits. Homeopathy penetrates deeply into the essence of a person, relieving any emotional and mental imbalance, and correcting the effects this imbalance has on the body, mind, and spirit. It is a totally holistic medicine.

Although homeopathy has been practiced for over several hundred years and is the medicine of choice in many parts of Europe, it is just now beginning to be accepted in the United States as a reliable alternative to conventional medicine. The remedies can be administered easily at home with positive results. They are safe and can be used by the entire family at any stage of life. Babies can ingest remedies through a bottle or their mother's milk. They can be used by young people and old people. They can be used throughout pregnancy and are effective for labor, delivery, and postpartum care.

Homeopathy is practiced today as it was originally conceived nearly 250 years ago by Dr. Samuel Hahnemann in Leipzig, Germany. Nothing has changed in homeopathic philosophy since that time. Thus as a medicine, it is anchored in solid ethical principles that are taught in the international homeopathic community and enforced.

This is not to say that homeopathy is old-fashioned with rigid guidelines. Just the opposite—it has adapted to the modern industrial world which is far different from Hahnemann's own era. Because people today are psychologically more complex and physically more dysfunctional than they were 200 years ago, homeopathic research has had to become more aware of the mental and emotional causes of physical symptoms. This is where homeopathy differs fundamentally from conventional medicine.

Homeopathy has been practiced in Europe, India, and Latin America for over two hundred years. It was and is still the preferred medicine of the royal families of Europe. In Britain, the royal family takes homeopathic remedies and advocates their use. Homeopathy is currently obtainable on the National Health Service as a medicine of choice.

In America homeopathy thrived until the early 1930s when the American Medical Association closed down the homeopathic medical schools and banned the practice of homeopathy in several states.

THE HISTORY OF HOMEOPATHY

Homeopathy was developed in Germany in the early 1700s by Dr. Samuel Hahnemann, a physician who became disillusioned with the medical practices of his day—he was losing more patients than he was saving. He therefore gave up his practice and began to earn his living by translating medical reports. In the course of his work, he came upon an article written by a physician named Cullen who proposed the use of cinchona bark as a cure for malaria. Curious about what the bark would do to him—he didn't have malaria—he swallowed a gram of cinchona and immediately experienced all the symptoms of malaria. He then reasoned that if a substance could create symptoms in a healthy person, it could cure the same symptoms in a sick person. He called his practice of healing homeopathy.

The strongest opposition to Hahnemann's practice and theories came from the pharmaceutical companies who were successful in running him out of Germany. In order to continue practicing, he moved to France. There Hahnemann found other physicians who shared his beliefs, and together they continued to examine many substances and tested their effect on healthy people.

In the beginning they studied folk remedies that had been used for thousands of years and then expanded their studies when Hahnemann discovered that some substances, though toxic in their material form, were not toxic when they were diluted, and, as a matter of fact, were more effective in extreme dilution. He never hesitated to try these medicines on himself and he recorded their effects. These observations are known as provings—they form the basis for the homeopathic materia medica.

As an example of a toxic substance becoming a remedy, there is a fascinating story about a great homeopath, Constantine Herring. He traveled to South America with his wife in search of substances that could be used as remedies. He heard about the most poisonous snake known to man, the bushmaster. After obtaining a live specimen, he told his wife to record all his symptoms after he first diluted the snake's venom and then ingested the solution. After he did so, he fell into a stupor and was unconscious for three days. However, his wife did record his symptoms, and we now have one of the most widely used, most powerful remedies in the entire materia medica, which is used today to treat jealousy, grief, delirium, hallucination, menopausal symptoms, and high septic states such as diphtheria. It is known as *Lachesis*.

Hahnemann lived and worked during the time of the great plagues that ravaged Europe. Entire populations of towns and villages were wiped out while doctors and pharmacists stood by, helpless. Hahnemann and his colleagues were able to save thousands of lives by noting the symptoms common to each plague and administering the similimum remedy. Allopathic doctors were losing nine out of ten patients, while Hahnemann and his colleagues were saving nine out of ten. This work of treating epidemics homeopathically is not generally recognized, but probably should be, considering the ever virulent flus striking large numbers of people and with autoimmune deficiency diseases on the increase.

Hahnemann made one other observation crucial in homeopathy: he observed that people vary in their response to an illness according to their temperament. This is the reason there are few prescriptive remedies. What works for one person may not work for another, though their symptoms might be similar. Homeopaths are taught to look for what is peculiar to each case. This is where homeopathy differs fundamentally from conventional medicine.

Today Hahnemann's work is still the backbone of homeopathy and the basis upon which good homeopaths practice.

THREE PRINCIPLES OF HOMEOPATHY
AS CONCEIVED BY HAHNEMANN

1. A medicine which in large doses produces the symptoms of a disease will in smaller doses cure the disease.

2. Through the process of extreme dilution, the medicine's curative properties are enhanced and all the poisonous or undesirable side effects are lost.

3. Homeopathic medicines are prescribed individually by the study of the whole person, according to that person's temperament and individual responses.

HOMEOPATHY'S SUCCESSES IN BRITAIN

I was trained as a classical homeopath in Britain, where homeopathy is recognized as an important field of medicine. Today the largest growing body of alternative practitioners in Britain are homeopaths: their ranks have grown over 400 percent in the past ten years. Homeopathy is practiced in clinics run and operated by the National Health Service. Private medical insurance believes in homeopathic treatment and pays for it. Businesses investing in homeopathy for their staff have found it dramatically reduced the number of sick days. Nursing homes are investigating homeopathy for gentle, cost-efficient treatment of the elderly, and midwives are studying the ways it can relieve the trauma of childbirth. Homeopathy is also gaining credibility and acceptance by the conventional medical community in Britain who are seeking reliable alternatives to conventional drugs and their side effects.

It has been discovered that over one-third of the patients in the National Health Hospitals in Britain suffer from iatrogenic diseases, brought on by conventional medical treatment, specifically drugs. It is important to look into a form of medicine which addresses all conditions without concurrent drug toxicity. Conventional medicine could then be used for what it does best: save lives, treat the terminally ill, perform necessary surgery, and look after basic health needs. Finding a proper place for each of these medicines is worthy of consideration by both allopathic and homeopathic practitioners.

WHAT CAN HOMEOPATHY DO FOR YOU?

In homeopathy we treat you, the individual, not the disease. We look at your physical, emotional, and mental symptoms to assess your case. We rely on the information we gather in interviews with you to help us prescribe a remedy that will address your condition and bring swift relief to your symptoms. We go over each area of your body and ask you to tell us how well you function. And if you can't express yourself, we ask those nearest you to tell us how you have been feeling and behaving. Oftentimes elderly people or very young children can't answer our questions and therefore we ask whoever takes care of them to describe their symptoms. We look for an underlying emotional cause of imbalance because we believe that your physical symptoms often mirror your emotional state.

We also look for family predisposition to conditions and diseases which may contribute to your case. We base our findings on simple facts, feelings, and experiences: how you feel and your emotional, mental, or physical response to your environment. These are all clues that will lead us to your remedy. We do not use machines to give us statistics, nor do we measure various systemic levels with tests.

WHAT ARE HOMEOPATHIC REMEDIES MADE OF?
WHAT CURES CAN YOU EXPECT?

Homeopathy's cures are numerous and its supporters great in number. Case after case of clinical evidence attest to its effectiveness. There are many people who were diagnosed as hopeless and given up by the allopathic medical community, who now experience full lives.

Homeopathic remedies are made from minerals, animals, and plants. They are very effective in the treatment of pets, dairy cows, goats, and cattle. Not only are vets using homeopathy on pets with excellent results, homeopaths are reportedly using it on wild animals who have been injured by environmental stress and pollution. Because there was evidence of an HIV-type disease decimating the dolphin population of the North Sea, several homeopaths set out in wetsuits to treat the dolphins with positive results. There is no placebo effect or psychological brainwashing possible when animals are treated with homeopathic remedies.

In order to diagnose animals, homeopaths rely on observation of their behavior. In order to diagnose people, homeopaths rely on interviews where clients report how they feel and how they respond to stress. Behavioral responses such as thirst, heat, cold, mobility, and lack of mobility must be observed. In those interviews we see what the Vital Force is doing and prescribe on that basis. We are looking for the whole range of symptoms that have upset the energetic economy so that we will understand how the remedy will work on subtle levels of the mind and emotions.

Homeopathy treats far more conditions than the medical community because it looks at the underlying emotional etiology. For example, there are no allopathic cures for bedwetting, fear, anxiety, or grief, whereas in homeopathy it is part of our practice to consider all aspects of human behavior. We also treat such conditions as asthma, heart disease, arthritis, cancer, and autoimmune deficiency diseases with success.

WHAT ARE PROVINGS?

We gather a picture of the effect of our remedies on healthy people and register these symptoms in our homeopathic *materia medica*. Each new symptom portrayed from a proving is added to our annals. This provides us with information about how a particular substance works. Our annals are based on over 250 years of experiments organized by categories. For instance, in a proving we note all the symptoms of the mind, head, face, throat, chest, respiration, heart, stomach, urination, bowels, sexual function, male and female differences, fevers, circulation, etc. This is the way a remedy portrait is developed. We want to know how a remedy works in its totality and what dimensions of the energetic economy it affects.

New provings are done annually on both old and new substances and, though our philosophy never changes, our *materia medica* is constantly expanding to meet the challenge of modern times.

All well-trained homeopaths are taught to read these provings. We base our evidence on the work of generations of practitioners who went before us who were meticulous in recording their clinical and laboratory findings that describe how a substance worked. Some of our remedies are presently being made from an original source over a hundred years old. What was used in homeopathy 250 years ago is still used to this day. We value all substances found in nature, and we examine them carefully to see how they work on the entire energetic economy, whether it is the physical, emotional, or mental realm.

It becomes very important to stay current with the remedies that are needed to shift the downward spiral of illness found in the population today. We are witness to more and more autoimmune deficiency diseases, attesting to some weakening in the vital force in a significant number of people. We also see a weakening in the human organism, apparent in people's increasing allergic reactions to external stimulation such as food additives, petrochemical pollution, and sexually transmitted diseases. How this general weakening will affect future generations in terms of health no one knows. Homeopaths feel that if we were to begin treatment today, it would take four generations before we would see a rise in the general health. We feel that it is our job to fortify the immune systems of our patients to resist any further decline.

Homeopathy looks deeply within the nature of the human psyche to rebalance the conditions that destroy and immobilize the will, that part of man/woman that helps us evolve and develop, that is required for getting on with our lives. Without a viable will, there is little that can be done to get a person's life back on track. Homeopaths treat people so that they can realistically assess their lives, and their will can be reengaged through conscious, good choices. This is healing that nurtures and fosters growth at all levels.

Unfortunately, too few people understand the profound healing that homeopathic medicine can bring. It works on so many levels of our energy system that, if used correctly, it can root out fears, phobias, and neuroses, and deal with physical problems as well. By finding the right homeopathic remedy, change becomes part of the natural evolutionary cycle of a person's life, and they are better able to develop on all levels.

In effect, homeopathic healing does not separate the deeper realms from the physical reality in which healing operates. We can see that a physical condition mirrors a state of mind, that when a person is suffering physically they may be undergoing a similar internal emotional process. This is reflected by the way they respond to a situation or a condition, even when those events happened a long time ago. What happens internally is also happening externally. The body acts as a reflection of our internal state and our emotions are reflected in our bodies.

Classical homeopathy believes in the use of one remedy at a time. We always wait to see how the remedy affects you on all levels before considering changing a remedy or increasing the potency. Conversely, if a remedy is working we do not change it. We are taught to be patient and watch for change on all levels.

A remedy may have a stronger effect on a mental level than on a physical level and vice versa. We need to see which realm is affected as well as how the remedy is rebalancing your symptoms. This takes time and observation.

WHAT WORKS FOR ONE PERSON
MAY NOT WORK FOR ANOTHER

Homeopaths are taught to look for what is peculiar to each case. This is what differentiates one remedy portrait from another and one person from another. If you question ten people about their headache symptoms, you will hear ten different responses. One person will feel a sharp pain in their left eye. Another person will feel a sharp pain in the back of their neck, while a third person will feel a sharp pain on the top of their head and have a stomachache. In homeopathy each of these headache symptoms would be treated with a different remedy. This approach has been proven the most positive and refined type of treatment. It has also made it difficult to be prescriptive.

Think of the different ways individuals react emotionally to a situation. For instance, in a tragedy, one person may be hysterical and become demanding and overwrought. Another person may feel incredibly sad and weep uncontrollably, wanting consolation and fearful of being alone. Still another may become silent and morose, and not wish to be with other people. Each person will react differently to the same situation. Homeopathy has remedies that address each one of these different conditions, even though each one is a response to the same external stimuli.

What is required in treatment is the ability to differentiate one emotional state from another, and the way one person responds to stimuli compared to another. How we determine our choice of remedies is based on observation, and the information we gather about these particular symptoms.

There are exceptions to this rule. Homeopathy *does* treat specific conditions when they are common to millions of people. For instance, there are only a handful of remedies for nosebleed. These work for most people. The same is true for cold symptoms and influenza.

GENETIC PREDISPOSITION

Treating genetic predisposition is one of the great gifts of homeopathy. Young people are encouraged to seek a qualified homeopath before they conceive. If constitutional treatment is given soon enough, it can prevent problems being handed down to the next generation. It can help particularly if there is a family history of cancer, heart disease, diabetes, or mental illness.

HOMEOPATHY IN THE WORKPLACE

I was hired by a large, multinational company in Britain as a qualified homeopath to help a team of sixteen creative people who worked in public relations. Their boss wanted them to function better both individually and with each other. Despite their wide variety of symptoms and conditions, they all responded well to treatment.

One person was completely depleted from three bouts of flu in a short period of time and four prescriptions of different antibiotics. She was beginning to show signs of autoimmune deficiency. Depressed and exhausted from the continuous travel that was necessary in her job, she was so worn out she often began weeping helplessly for no apparent reason. She wanted to quit her job. However, within a week of homeopathic treatment she had new vitality and stamina for her work at home and on the job.

The way the treatment succeeded with the entire team was interesting. The group had one day for orientation, in which they learned what homeopathy was, how it worked, and how it could benefit their minor and major health problems. I gave them first aid kits and taught them how to use them. Opportunely, on the first day of orientation, a man tripped over a lead wire on the floor and fell down. Bruised and upset, he was given *Arnica* 6x from the homeopathic first aid kit and within minutes was free of aches and pains. It was direct evidence for him and the rest of the group. Convinced of the value of homeopathy, the team began to use their first aid kits for minor problems. And, when I offered them a session for constitutional treatment as an option, fifteen out of the sixteen people accepted.

As for the group as a whole, I read their medical histories before I met them. I then held one hour interviews with each person in which they discussed their health issues and the effect of stress on their lives. I gave first aid remedies to those people who were suffering from acute problems like cold, flu, and post-viral fatigue. Within twenty-four hours they responded positively and returned to work with renewed energy. The other cases, which were constitutional in nature, took approximately one month to show a significant response.

All the members of the team reported that they felt better emotionally and that their work was more focused. Six weeks later, everyone reported they had improved in health, mental outlook, and emotional stability, even though they had been under more stress than usual with project deadlines. They all agreed that they had handled the stress very well. Some had made decisions about their future and had applied for new jobs with their employer. They all felt they could manage challenges with new energy. All had experienced some degree of change, and all responded positively to treatment.

Because of this experience, I learned that homeopathy has a major place in the workforce. It can make a difference in the productivity and creativity of a significant number of people, even though I maintained an individual approach to each person's conditions.

This team was composed of basically healthy young adults (under 45). They were overworked and underpaid for their time and energy, and they were rundown. Yet they responded within six weeks to treatment in astounding ways. They took their kits home and used them for themselves and their families and friends. Within a few months they were familiar with how homeopathy worked for them and they all attested to their sense of health and well-being from using it.

Looking at the pace of our lives it has become apparent we don't have time for long recoveries and lingering symptoms. Homeopathy can resolve many core issues. It addresses the emotions and rebalances the system so that healing can take place on deep and profound levels. It works so smoothly in most cases that it holds a promise of health that few medicines can make. It gives people their lives back, without creating a dependency on medicine or on the practitioner.

How Does Homeopathy Work?

This medicine works differently from conventional medicine. Its philosophy that less is more may be confusing to you. Let's look at how homeopathy works.

First, homeopathy requires you to be aware of your symptoms and the aspects of your condition that are specific to you. Let us assume you have a headache that plagues you regularly. A homeopath would want to know how regularly you experience this headache. Is it periodic in its occurrence?

Whatever is unique to your condition needs to be noted. For instance, you may dislike going out in bright light when you have a headache, or you may desire cold drinks, or you may lose your appetite when you are feeling poorly. Whatever you can note that will distinguish your symptoms is important for finding the remedy that will help you.

If you take an aspirin for your headache, be assured your headache will return when a similar stress provokes it again. In homeopathy when the underlying cause is addressed, in many cases the susceptibility to the problem is completely eliminated. This is one reason it is so effective; it goes to the core of things to reestablish balance and harmony.

But before you can be given a remedy that will eliminate your headache and stop it from reoccurring, it is essential to dissect its components and analyze the manner in which it operates. Every aspect of how you feel when this headache or any other symptom occurs needs to be looked at. When this information is collated, a remedy is carefully chosen that contains the totality of your symptoms in its remedy portrait. It is then prescribed for you.

Remember, arriving at the right remedy is only as good as the information you give the homeopath. To simply say you have a headache means nothing to a homeopath. Because it is such an individual medicine, it demands that therapeutic guidelines be followed carefully for positive results. A homeopath needs to ask, What are the qualities of your condition? Where does it hurt? Is the pain in the front, side, back of your body? How would you describe the pain? Is it dull, aching, sharp, throbbing, constricting? What else is going on physically, emotionally, and mentally? Are you feeling irritable, sad, anxious, fearful? Are you thirsty or not thirsty at all? Can you think clearly, do you want fresh air, or do you want to lie down? These are the things that help determine which remedy suits your condition.

It is important to clarify symptoms when searching for a remedy. There are simple keynote symptoms that help differentiate one remedy from another. For instance, we may want to know what provoked the headache, and how you react when you have a headache. Besides the symptoms above, do you feel better or worse for eating? Do you crave milk, sweets, or some other food? Are you constipated when you have a headache? Does your stomach ache or do your legs feel weak? What makes you feel better or worse?

These concomitant symptoms will help you get the right remedy. They may seem unimportant to you, but they can make a difference to your well-being. It is important to pay attention to your temperament. Are you irritable, angry, sad, frustrated, depressed? All these symptoms are signs that will lead you to your remedy. Often a remedy will have levels of irritability, anxiety, fear, sadness, or apathy which go along with its physical symptoms. They are all noted in the *materia medica*.

When you describe your symptoms ask yourself how you feel emotionally. It will assist you in arriving at a remedy that works for you. We are too accustomed to thinking of medicine as a cure for our physicality; we do not see the accompanying emotional picture.

A recent case in point is of a woman who was moving from her home. She was surrounded by clutter and felt angry that her son was not helping her. The weather was very hot and she, a natural redhead, was very flushed. She had a headache, was not thirsty, but the top of her head was throbbing. She was given a *Belladonna* 6x and within a few minutes her color returned to normal, the headache had disappeared, and she realized how angry she was at her son for leaving her with a mess. This was quick healing. It not only brought relief, it brought self-awareness.

Whatever state you are in, the remedy which works for you will match your internal state. It will address every level of your unbalance. It not only addresses a physical symptom and leaves you in an internal state of irritability and agitation. It works at the core of your being and rebalances you at every level. It helps you to move forward in your life while eliminating the underlying factors that create the imbalance in the first place.

In homeopathy there are no biochemical statistics that will prove *how* the similimum remedy stimulates your Vital Force to respond. We do know from many trials that the remedies work when we look at the deeper mental and emotional factors that go along with the physical symptoms. We don't know how they work.

If you went to a homeopath soon after a relationship broke up, complaining of a chronic sore throat and headache, you would be asked about your grief, how you handle the expression of your feelings, and what you feel is still unresolved in that relationship. Your response would help the homeopath determine what remedy would be best suited to you right now.

You may come back to see the homeopath with the same exact sore throat a year later. But you are different now from the way you were when you saw her before. You have recovered from your grief and are now suffering from feelings of suppressed anger with your boss for not listening to your good ideas. It is obvious that one of your areas of susceptibility is your throat and issues of communication, but your emotional etiology is completely different this time. So the remedy that would help you with your throat symptoms and your feelings of loss would be different the second time. On your original visit your condition was caused by unexpressed grief; the second condition was caused by unexpressed anger. Though the same area is affected, the emotions are different and so are the remedies.

Homeopaths are now better able to follow scientific guidelines for how change occurs in the physical economy, and they are performing double-blind studies on the ways in which the remedies work. Homeopathy takes time to bring about healing, and it is particularly slow for long-term chronic conditions. For these we give a remedy, wait, and watch to see how you respond. However, it works miraculously for first-aid problems and acute conditions.

We measure only clinical results and evident symptom alleviation. Remedies are never repeated when the condition has cleared up. The homeopathic definition of health is not limited to the absence of disease or the relief of symptoms. Emotional stability, mental clarity, and well-functioning lives are also a part of the spectrum of health. We measure results by looking at quality of life in every case. We don't say you are healed because your ulcer is healed. We suggest that you may wish to treat other areas of susceptibility that limit your effectiveness in living the life you say you want. We suggest you explore some of the other dimensions in your life where you are not happy or fulfilled, and then treat those homeopathically. We strive for complete balance and wholeness in our patients. This is what homeopathy can offer to people. It is wonderful for people who are going through times of change and transformation.

Few people, outside of homeopaths and patients, know how deep homeopathy can go and how it can restore health and vitality. Our definition of health is broad. It includes supporting your capacity to live harmoniously. This medicine helps people adapt to change, and to undergo internal transformation that aligns them with their higher purpose in life.

THE VITAL FORCE IN MANKIND

Homeopathy addresses the life principle in each person. The Vital Force is that aspect of all things which is alive and vital and acts as the internal guiding principle to regulate every bodily function. It is also known as the immune system. It controls your heartbeat, reduces a fever when you are ill, and lets you know you are hungry, thirsty, irritable, sad, or happy. This part of you is shared with all things living. It does not exist in us when we die. It is that part of us that responds to life; it becomes irritated, it grieves, suffers, laughs, delights, loves, and is adaptable to change. This is the part that when it is chilled produces a fever to compensate. When it is unhappy, it creates symptoms of stress and irritability. It controls all vital functions at every level of existence and acts in all systems of the body to produce symptoms we can see and treat. In homeopathy we believe that all symptoms are there to give us a picture of the levels of health or dysfunction in a person. Symptoms are signs of how the Vital Force is functioning.

Homeopaths are taught to read, see, and hear the signs of the Vital Force. We know that symptoms can be addressed with a remedy which contains similar symptoms in its portrait as your Vital Force is displaying. In response to a remedy, the Vital Force once again assumes a level of harmony and well-being.

The stronger the individual's Vital Force, the stronger their symptoms. Weak symptoms indicate a compromised Vital Force. Therefore, a healthy organism will have very strong symptoms when it is out of balance. You see this in healthy children who have high fevers and strong reactions to infection. Paradoxically, you have to be healthy to be very ill. This is a difficult concept to accept if you are not familiar with homeopathic thinking.

People with weak immunities don't have enough vitality to become ill. When a person gets a cold after taking a remedy, it is considered a sign of health, rather than weakness. It shows that the Vital Force has been stimulated and detoxification is beginning. It also means mental symptoms may move to the physical level to be expressed.

The strength and vitality of the Vital Force is apparent in new life, and when there is an imbalance it is instantly apparent. Healthy babies and young children become ill quickly. Their symptoms must also be treated promptly with a remedy that contains a similar degree of vitality in its portrait. Delicate constitutions require delicate remedies and a gentle potency.

Very ill and terminally ill patients do not have strong symptoms. They have a diminished Vital Force, not strong enough to produce vibrant symptoms. What they experience is a general malaise or lack of reactive powers. The treatment given them needs to be a very gentle dilution, not something that is going to upset their delicately balanced system. Homeopathic remedies are chosen for their similimum qualities and for the reactive force of the potency used.

POTENTIZATION

Potentization refers to the level a homeopathic remedy is diluted. Each state of dilution is called a potency. The higher the potency, the stronger the remedy, and the deeper its realm of action. The higher the potency, the more the remedy works at mental and emotional levels and the longer its effect is felt. Some remedies can last up to a year with one single dose.

What this means in terms of treatment is that if you have a headache you would take a dose of a 6x (or 6 dilution) of the remedy selected to match your symptoms. You may need to repeat this remedy several times during the day. When the headache is alleviated, you stop taking the remedy. If, however, you were attempting to stop your susceptibility to headaches altogether, as in the case of chronically occurring headaches or migraine, you would take the similimum remedy in a high potency of perhaps a 200c (200 dilutions), and you would take it only once and *not* repeat it. In attempting to rebalance the body, this remedy could be effective for several months. It is given only one time, and the dynamic effects go on for weeks and weeks.

Potency is generally done is incremental shifts of 3, 6, 12, 30, 200, 1000, 10,000, 50,000 and 100,000. The "x" refers to dilution in decimals. This means that the substance is diluted in ten drops of water and alcohol. A "c" dilution refers to a dilution in one hundred drops of water and alcohol. They are similar in their effect with the "c" being slightly stronger in higher potency. Remedies are often potentized in "x" dilutions under 12 potencies. After that they are potentized in "c" dilutions.

The rule of thumb is that when you take a remedy of low potency of 6x and under, you treat quickly and easily. The realm of action is generally physical and does not have a deep or long-term effect on the emotions or mental attitudes.

For first aid treatment the remedies are recommended at 6x, and occasionally 30c for serious conditions. These can be purchased at health food stores and from homeopathic pharmacies.

For higher dilution it is recommended that you see a homeopath for treatment. Once you get into higher potencies you need a well-trained homeopath because expertise is important at this level. Self-treatment with high potencies is *not* encouraged.

HOW A REMEDY IS MADE

A remedy is made in the following manner. A substance is taken from nature and either boiled or triturated (crushed) to produce a supply which can be made into a tincture. This is known as the mother tincture and is symbolized in homeopathy with this symbol (ø). This means that the substance is in its most basic state before dilution.

If you were to take *Hawthorn*, for instance, which is used in the treatment of heart conditions, you would begin to make the remedy by boiling up the leaves, flowers, and bark taken from a Hawthorn tree at the time the flower was in optimal bloom in early spring. This is when the Vital Force of this plant is at its strongest, when it contains more energy than at any other time. Eventually with enough boiling you would produce a heavily concentrated serum. This serum is used in herbalism just as it is to make herbal tinctures. In homeopathic remedies the process begins by making the first dilution. This is done by taking one single drop of the serum and adding it to a mixture of ten drops of water and alcohol. You now have what is known in homeopathy as the first dilution (1x). Then if you take one drop of this mixture and add it to another ten drops of water and alcohol, you have the second dilution. This process continues of taking one drop of solution and placing it in a solution of water and alcohol until you have the number of dilutions required.

REPETITION OF A REMEDY

Normally, higher potencies are not repeated, while low potencies of 6x are repeated often. This is because the higher the potency the more dynamic the medicine and the more powerful its realm of influence.

A general rule of thumb is that if a low potency remedy is repeated three times in a short period of time and has not altered the symptoms for which it was intended, it is not the similimum and you need to choose another remedy. This applies to first aid and acute cases. Chronic treatment takes much longer to assess. It is believed that if you have the similimum remedy the potency is not as important as the remedy itself. Selecting a remedy carefully will alleviate your symptoms.

Lower potencies are very effective and quick to address symptoms. It is not normal for a patient to need more than a couple of doses of a remedy to have their first aid symptoms alleviated.

For instance, if you had a nosebleed and you saw in the first aid kit that *Ferrum Phos.* was the suitable remedy, you would take one dose of a 6x and wait five minutes. If the bleeding had slowed down but was not completely gone you would take one more dose. If this completely stopped the bleeding you would not take any more of the remedy. If you were to continue to do so you might create the condition you were trying to stop, in this case a nosebleed.

Remedies are taken only while the symptoms last. You do not take a remedy if there is not a symptom. This is important!

If you feel you want a higher potency for a remedy, remember that it is more important to get the similimum remedy than to worry about the potency. A low potency of a remedy (this is usually considered to be 3x, 6x, 12c) can be extremely effective, even if it is necessary to repeat over a period of time.

A middle level potency (a 30c, for instance) can be given once, even twice a day, for a short duration of up to three days and left to act. This level of potency can treat chronic symptoms very effectively, and is good for mild, chronic conditions such as sinusitis, constipation, or symptoms that are irritating but not undermining to your health.

OVERDOSING

Be careful. Don't overdose on a remedy. It is common in our culture to think that more is better. In homeopathy the rule is that less is more. Less can transform your energy and health to a very high degree. You do not need to pour a lot of medicine into your body for it to work. What you have to do is get the right remedy and let it stimulate your Vital Force back into balance.

When you do have the right remedy, proceed cautiously and wait to see how it affects you. If you have a headache, for instance, and you decide that the portrait of *Bryonia* suits your symptoms, you would take one 6x (not two as are prescribed by the commercial pharmaceutical companies who are trying to sell more bottles of their product) and wait for half an hour to see if your headache went away. If it did you would not need to repeat the remedy. What you are putting into your body is a frequency of vibration. If you take one small pill or a bathtub full of pills you are still only receiving that one frequency of vibration.

If your headache did not go away, but was only partially relieved, you would take a second pill and let it work. If after half an hour, you had no symptoms at all, you could take a third pill. It is not advisable to take more than five doses of a remedy in a day. If you feel that you need to do this, you most likely do not have the right remedy.

If you put a lot of different remedies into your body and none of them worked, you should give some thought to seeing a homeopath to discuss your case. A professionally trained and qualified practitioner is better able to assess your case. Moreover, they have a variety of remedies at their disposal. Also, the practitioner may be better able to access your case in terms of familial predisposition, stress-related factors, and past medical history. They are trained to evaluate your case in the light of many contributory causes, which you may not be able to see.

A THEORETICAL CASE

Let's look at a theoretical case so that you can see how treatment works. Let's use the case of the grief-stricken patient we discussed early on in this chapter. He was upset over the loss of a relationship. He is shocked and does not cry or respond to this situation, but swallows his grief, feeling it is far too painful to feel. His temperament does not allow him to express feelings openly and he can grieve only in private. Nevertheless, he is hurt. His grief congests his energy because he holds on to his grief. After a period of time he develops symptoms which are not normal for him. He eats too many sweets that stick in his throat and he has trouble swallowing. He gets a headache that feels like a nail is being driven into his head, and he feels irritable, moody, and incommunicative. If he doesn't realize these are not normal, they will become more acute until he's forced to pay attention. This is how the Vital Force is signaling him that he is not in harmony with his deep self. It is creating a portrait of grief for him to see in the hope that healing can happen. A homeopath notes these sensations and symptoms, and matches them against the mental, emotional, and physical symptoms displayed in various remedies in the *materia medica*.

In homeopathy we define disease as separation from the self. When this happens we create symptoms that tell astute observers trained to observe symptoms that something is not right. These symptoms of grief linger and somaticize in the body as pain or dysfunction and they do not improve, even with aspirin or drugs. This is more than a physical case, though many of the symptoms are on the physical plane. The person then decides to visit a homeopath. Let's look at how the procedure unfolds, and how a remedy is found to help this person feel better.

VISITING THE HOMEOPATH

After a few weeks of continuing symptoms, he calls to make an appointment. The homeopath sends a family history form to be returned before the consultation. On the first visit the homeopath has scheduled an hour and a half for the consultation which involves answering questions and talking about oneself. The homeopath wants to know all about this person, how he feels about things, his emotional response to situations, what he likes, what he dislikes, what he fears, what he loves.

Questions are asked about his general health in all the systems of the body, including sleep patterns, and other cycles such as menstruation. Questions are asked about appetite and what he likes and dislikes in food and drink. The way in which he responds is observed. It is noted if he is anxious, aggressive, closed, or open. When the consultation is completed, the homeopath may tell the person that a remedy will be sent to him with clear instructions. He will be asked to make note of how he feels after taking the remedy, and to call the homeopath with questions.

In this hypothetical case, after taking the remedy the headache completely disappears within a few days and cycles start to readjust; sleep and dreams are deeper. The craving for sweets disappears as does the lump in the throat. At some point the emotions may be engaged and the grief appropriately expressed in tears. Within a short time he feels like his old self. This treatment reflects the holistic nature of the medicine and the way in which a person is treated for his mind/body/spirit.

CAN HOMEOPATHY WORK FOR YOU?

The degree of healing this medicine can provide you throughout your life is well worth investigating. You may find it worthwhile to get a consultation and find out if your condition can be treated and if you can achieve higher levels of health and vitality by taking homeopathy.

It is important to ask questions if there is something you don't understand about your treatment. Ask your homeopath about what is involved in your particular case. The more responsibility you are willing to take for your health, the better your treatment will be for you. It is important to get as much information as possible. Be sure that you fully understand the procedure and the length of time your condition needs for healing. Ask questions, keep track of how you feel, and note the changes in your body, mind, and spirit. Read books, ask questions, and take responsibility for what you want to see happen to your general well-being.

WHAT CAN AND CANNOT BE TREATED HOMEOPATHICALLY?

Of course, homeopathy works best on people who are receptive to it. It can, however, be used on the elderly, infants, and animals who may have no say in their treatment. It works best in someone who is not taking conventional or herbal medicine. Each form of medicine has its unique realm of action. The only way a homeopath can observe your reaction to a remedy is to have you as drug free as possible. So it is suggested you do not mix treatments with other alternative or allopathic medicine, unless it is essential for your health.

If you are presently taking a medicine that suppresses symptoms and take a homeopathic remedy, you create confusion and conflict in your body. If you are taking cortisone or antibiotics, for instance, these powerful drugs will create a picture that may make it difficult to know what symptoms are true to your constitution and which symptoms are created by the drugs. Homeopathy can work when people are heavily medicated, though it is not ideal. Aggravation may arise and create discomfort for the patient and confusion for the practitioner. Even the birth control pill, highly suppressive of the life force, can make deep constitutional treatment slower and less effective.

Homeopathy is generally slow but effective in constitutional and chronic cases. First aid treatment is very responsive, and because the potency is kept very low the chance of aggravating the body is minimal.

If you wish to treat a specific condition it is best to understand that homeopathic treatment is addressed to the whole person. It does not treat a disease because that is a label. It treats the totality of symptoms that create your distress and imbalance. A condition has other components that are part of an overall picture of imbalance such as feelings and thoughts.

If you have doubts about the effectiveness of homeopathy, please consult a homeopath in your area. He or she can suggest a consultation where you can talk over your case and inquire as to whether homeopathy would be an effective treatment.

In terminal diseases homeopathy is a wonderful gift. As it promotes quality of life, it helps relieve symptoms that can be painful and uncomfortable. It can allow a person to end their time with dignity, minimal discomfort, and clarity of mind. Many people fear death and some of the remedies used to treat the terminally ill will help make the experience less fearful. It can ease the distress of those who are nursing the ill and dying as well.

Any time a person is in extreme conditions that stretch their emotions and nerves, homeopathy can ease their symptoms. It is excellent for major life changes, in childbirth, for teething infants, toddlers, youth, adults, and the elderly. It can treat asthma, eczema, and the variety of childhood diseases that make parenting a full-time job. It can help adolescents deal with this major life change, and help regulate growth, relieve acne, and other changes that accompany adolescence. It is excellent for young adults to boost job confidence and increase the possibility of success.

Homeopathy is the best ticket for aging I know. It can help regulate menopause so that it becomes a time when new options and possibilities can manifest. It can also treat bone density, ligament weakness, joint stiffness, and calcium depletion without putting dangerous drugs into the body. In fact, it is so effective in menopause that hot flashes and night sweats disappear. In short, it has been used to aid aging so that the wisdom of elders can be preserved along with a strong and viable physical body to support the spirit.

In extreme cases of mental disease where medication is necessary, homeopathy has been used to reduce episodes of violence, hysteria, and acting out. Because it addresses the mental and emotional aspects of the personality, it brings order promptly to anyone who is distressed.

Homeopathy has been used in the treatment of autistic and Alsperger's disease where cognitive disorders inhibit socialization. And it has been used in mental hospitals to reduce violent outbursts without having to medicate patients heavily.

It is less effective when a person is on medications that suppress vital function, although in drug dependency of any kind this medicine works to stimulate the Vital Force again.

Homeopathy is a complete medicine. It is designed to treat the individual and not the disease. It is effective because it triggers the natural vitality of the person to respond holistically, bringing about balance and harmony over a period of time on all levels. In the case of first aid this readjustment can happen quickly. In deeper constitutional treatment the rebalancing can take a period of time.

Homeopathic First Aid Remedies

HOW TO LOCATE THE REMEDY FOR YOU

You must choose the remedy which most closely matches your symptoms. Notice as many characteristics of your condition as possible and match them with the symptoms noted in the remedy. Note the location and the site affected to see if they match the location in the remedy picture. Pay attention to what makes you feel better: lying in a certain position, or if you are better or worse from such things as pressure, touch, bending, moving your head or back, in fresh air, being tightly clothed.

Other symptoms, such as your emotional state, help you to find the similimum remedy. Self-observation is crucial in treatment. It isn't enough to say you have a pain here or there. How do you feel? Are you irritable, sad, angry; do you despair of recovery, anticipate an event, or are you frightened? These emotional keynotes make a difference in determining your remedy. They go along with the specific physical questions: Where is it? What makes it feel better or worse? Which side is it on, etc.

So, in locating your first aid remedy, pay attention to yourself or the person you are treating. Homeopathic remedies have no side effects. If you do not choose the right remedy, you will not experience any change in your symptoms. If you fail to note what goes on with your case you may fail to achieve the healing you seek. The remedy needs to be carefully chosen in order to be effective. Homeopathic first aid is gentle and very effective when you get the right remedy and you can be assured it will work for you. The remedies in this book are recommended for first aid and injuries only. They are not recommended for deeper chronic or constitutional care. When dealing with acute first aid conditions, the remedies need to be precisely matched to the patient's symptoms. Read the symptoms over carefully and determine which remedy suits your condition.

1. Please note the *location*, which is the exact position of the symptoms.

2. Pay attention to the *sensations*, which are the feelings you experience, such as heat, cold, dizziness, pain. Note what type of pain it is, such as sharp, throbbing, aching, dull.

3. Please be aware of the *modalities*, which are whatever makes the symptoms feel better or worse.

4. If it is possible to be aware of the *cause* of the symptoms this may be very helpful in finding the remedy you need. Your emotional state could be the result of a stressful or unhappy situation.

HOW TO TAKE THE REMEDIES

There are several ways to take a remedy. The easiest way is in pill form. Take one pill, place it under your tongue, and let it dissolve. Many bottles from homeopathic pharmacies require you to take two or more pills. There is no need to waste your supply of remedies when one pill does the trick.

As the remedy dissolves under your tongue, avoid water or food for ten minutes before and after you take the remedy. If you need to repeat the remedy, keep it out of the sunlight or away from strongly scented things like perfume or tobacco while you wait to repeat it. These will weaken the strength of the remedy and its effect. It is suggested that remedies be kept in cool, dark places while they are not in use. They should also be kept away from strongly scented things like camphor, lavender, eucalyptus, perfume, essential oils, detergent, or tobacco.

Another way of taking a remedy is with powder sachets. They are placed directly on the tongue. This is the way they are sold in homeopathic pharmacies in Europe, specifically in Belgium and France. You may come across a pharmacy where they are prepared in this way. Drops are sometimes used but often require that the bottle be shaken several times before each treatment. If you have a liquid remedy it can also be sniffed. This has proved effective for many people who are very responsive to remedies.

TREATING BABIES AND INFANTS

For babies or small children you can do the following: if you are treating a nursing baby, have the mother take the pill and pass the remedy to the child through her milk. It is a direct way of treating and there is no time lapse once the mother has ingested the pill. For a bottle-fed baby, let the remedy dissolve in the bottle of milk, water, or juice. It is important to remember that it is not a question of quantity, it is the contact with the remedy that is important. Give the baby the amount of fluid it cares to drink. It is not a matter of how much fluid is ingested. What is important is that the fluid make contact with the baby's mouth.

In an emergency, place the remedy under the upper lip of the child and hold the lip down for at least ten seconds.

Homeopathic remedies can work promptly to get into the bloodstream. The medication will be absorbed from the coated pill. The child does not need to ingest the pill, only to have contact with it for ten seconds. Remember, do not eat or drink anything for at least ten minutes prior to or after the remedy. The remedy must get into the blood without any interference as quickly as possible.

If the remedy is working and needs to be repeated, you can take it again within two minutes for an emergency, but no more than three doses more. If it is not an emergency, repeat after twenty minutes to half an hour for up to three doses. When the remedy begins to work and be effective, spread out the doses until the symptoms disappear. Once they are gone, stop giving the remedy altogether. It is meant to be used only while the symptom lasts.

HOW DO YOU KNOW THAT YOU HAVE THE RIGHT REMEDY?

You know that you have given the correct remedy because symptoms begin to disappear and you feel better. It is a very pragmatic form of medicine. If it is not working, you do not have the right remedy.

Check again to make sure that the symptoms match the picture of the remedy listed in the *materia medica* at the back of the book. Check again on the following: Are you thirsty? Do you feel better lying down or sitting up? Do you crave warmth or do you crave cold fresh air? These are the points that can make the difference in selecting the right remedy for the case. The wrong remedy has no effect. The right remedy alleviates the symptoms you are treating quickly and efficiently.

ARE THERE ANY SIDE EFFECTS?

There are no side effects in homeopathy. In first aid you can expect instant results, such as an end to a hemorrhage or a headache. There are no half measures with homeopathy; either you have the similimum and it works or you have not chosen the appropriate remedy.

Chemical drugs have so-called side effects. These destabilize the body and cause the kidneys, liver, and stomach to process heavy acid that harms the delicate tissues and organs of the body. In homeopathy you can experience aggravation when taking a constitutional remedy. For instance, in order for the body to detoxify from congestion you may develop a rash, have a bout of loose bowels, or experience a headache briefly while the body readjusts itself to regain balance. This can be experienced as mild discomfort. It is not a side effect and it is not damaging in any way. It is the result of the imbalance that already exists.

CAN YOU CAUSE HARM OR DAMAGE TAKING THE WRONG REMEDY?

No. The wrong remedy is released through the urine and leaves no trace of any kind. There are stories of children getting into first aid kits and taking a variety of remedies with absolutely no side effects. When the remedy is not the similimum, it does not act. It is not a chemical or herbal potion. It is an energetic substance that needs to match the portrait of your specific symptoms in order to restore balance.

Remember, the substance that is made into a remedy has a picture of symptoms that should match your symptoms. When you take a remedy it relieves those symptoms. It does nothing else to you.

WHAT TO DO AFTER THE FIRST AID TREATMENT

If you feel that this form of medicine works for you, and you want to know if it can do more to help you in a general way, visit a homeopath. You can also take courses in first aid, take home study programs, and read books that will help you understand the nature of homeopathy and how it can help, balance, and bring relief to you and your family.

CAN YOU TAKE HOMEOPATHIC AND REGULAR MEDICINE?

Homeopathy is a complete medicine in itself. It is life enhancing and does not suppress symptoms as conventional medicine does. Taking the two together can cause disruption in your general health and is not encouraged.

In conventional medicine, symptoms are suppressed—they are pushed deeper into the body. For instance, in conventional medicine when you have a skin problem such as eczema, cortisone is given for relief of the itching and redness. Cortisone pushes the symptoms deeper into the body. The next thing you know, you experience joint aches and pains where the toxins, once on the surface of the body, are now deeper in the body. If more medicine is administered for this, systemic symptoms appear indicating weakened and debilitated organs. Eventually, after prolonged use of allopathic drugs, weakness forms in the tissues of the heart and liver. The system is so overdosed with drugs that it weakens and breaks down completely. The drugs have compromised the general immunity of the patient.

Homeopathy, because it is an energetic medicine, strives to build the energetic economy and revitalize the body. This means that it strengthens the immune system and rebalances the Vital Force. It does this by pushing symptoms up to the surface. It frees the deep organs of toxins, so that they may function properly. We want symptoms to move from the deep core out to the surface.

When you take a deep-acting constitutional homeopathic remedy it will bring symptoms out to the surface of the body. We anticipate rashes and discharges, which strengthen the core of a person and aid in the detoxification of deep tissue. We find that people generally feel better when this happens, even when they may experience external symptoms. We believe that toxins and impurities are better out of the body than congesting and weakening the system internally. So we never suppress rashes; we soothe them with homeopathic ointments, and work to detoxify the deeper organs. We want toxins out onto the surface of the body, away from the core, where they can cause severe disruption of health.

We do not encourage the mixture of allopathic, herbal, or ayurvedic medicine, or acupuncture while on a remedy. It creates confusion in the body and is not effective. In order to see how your system reacts to remedies it is best to be free of medication and off supplements. If you feel weak and debilitated, we want to see that picture and treat it. When there is a condition on the skin we know that it will eventually be relieved. We know that when you develop a skin symptom something deep within the body is discharging toxins. We would not do anything to suppress this symptom, other than see that you were comfortable. But in the case of eczema or acne, for instance, we treat the deep inner organs to establish balance so that the skin symptoms clear up.

In conventional medicine you would be given a remedy to stop any skin irritation. It is our experience in homeopathy that when this is done, symptoms internalize and disease patterns take hold from toxic congestion of the cells. When asthma develops after treating eczema or a skin rash with cortisone, you have begun the process of immunosuppression, which eventually weakens and debilitates you.

Conventional medicine acts in the opposite way from homeopathy. However, if a person is on medicine which is life sustaining and important for the treatment of a chronic and serious condition, we would give our medicine in gentle doses that would not conflict with their medicine. For instance, in the treatment of diabetes, we would never suggest that a patient come off insulin. That would create such imbalance in the body that it could be life threatening. We would use very dilute forms of homeopathic medicine, called LM potency, and stop it immediately if the patient exhibited a stressful reaction to it. We try to stimulate the Vital Force to reactivate itself.

Medicines, such as cortisone, antibiotics, and birth control pills are suppressive. When you give homeopathic remedies along with these you can create an aggravation where the Vital Force wants to rid itself of the suppressed symptoms. Conflict develops in the physical body with one medicine trying to push symptoms down and another trying to bring them out. Also, the remedies do not work as effectively because of the level of suppression caused by these powerful drugs.

ARE REMEDIES ADDICTIVE OR HARMFUL? DO THEY HAVE HARMFUL EFFECTS IF YOU TAKE TOO MANY?

No. Homeopathic remedies are not addictive in any way, nor can you do any harm to the system if you take too many pills. As I mentioned, there are stories of children getting into homeopathic remedies and having no ill effects at all. A remedy needs to be the right one to have any effect, and if this is what the child needs it will work on their system. If it is not what they need it will not have any effect at all. This is what makes homeopathy such an excellent and affirming medicine.

It is important to stop taking a homeopathic remedy as soon as your symptoms cease. Otherwise your body may reproduce the symptoms it has just eliminated.

This is another way we differ from allopathic medicine. We do not give courses of remedies. We give them and take them for only the duration of the symptoms. When the symptoms cease it is time to stop the remedy.

WHAT ARE BACH FLOWER ESSENCES AND WHAT DO THEY DO?

The Bach remedies are made from distilled water and flowers. They work to stabilize the emotions. Bach remedies capture the emotion essence of each flower. The flower essence provides an emotional stability that calms, soothes, and balances the nerves, and can be very useful, particularly in emergencies for fear and anxiety.

The best known of all Bach remedies is Rescue Remedy. It is made of five different flower essences and brings instant relief to many first aid symptoms. Once you have seen its effectiveness you wouldn't want to be without it. Many people carry it in their handbags, in the glove compartments of their cars, and use it for a multitude of symptoms. It can be purchased wherever you buy homeopathic remedies.

When using Rescue Remedy it is suggested to dilute it. Take two drops of the tincture and add it to a quarter-cup of water. Sip it over a period of time. It will help soothe the nerves and ease the spirit and can bring instant relief to disturbed nerves. It can be used straight out of the bottle in serious emergencies, but it is best used diluted.

In the following list of therapeutic conditions you can also use a Bach flower remedy to accompany the homeopathic remedy and color essence.

HOMEOPATHIC COLOR REMEDIES: WHAT ARE THEY AND WHAT PURPOSE DO THEY SERVE?

I developed these remedies. They have an affinity with energy centers in the body, known as Chakras. The way color remedies work is to cool down areas that are hot, congested, and inflamed by using the cool colors, or by heating the areas of the body which are deprived of blood and need energy with hot colors. They are gentle, safe, and effective. For first aid treatments, always use the 6x potency. Color remedies go a long way to revitalize your energy. They can soothe a headache, alleviate cramps, congestion, and constipation. Should you desire to read more about them see *Homeopathic Color Remedies*, published by The Crossing Press.

You can use color remedies along with the homeopathic and Bach remedy if you like.

Note: To effect deep healing of tissue and pathology, take the homeopathic remedy first and then the Bach and color remedies.

First Aid Conditions

ABDOMINAL PAINS

This refers to all stomach pains that arise from eating, from fear, anxiety, or for any other reason.

When food feels like a stone in the pit of the stomach and the patient feels better after resting (the discomfort is accompanied with a bilious feeling and a slight headache):

Homeopathic Remedy: **Bryonia** — and/or

Bach Remedy: **Rescue Remedy**

Color Remedy: **Yellow**

When the stomach is bloated with accompanying gas after light intake of food:

Homeopathic Remedy: **Lycopodium** — and/or

Bach Remedy: **Cerato**

Color Remedy: **Yellow**

When there is gas and colic after eating and drinking alcohol:

Homeopathic Remedy: **Nux Vom** — and/or

Bach Remedy: **Vine**

Color Remedy: **Indigo**

ABRASIONS

Clean the wound with a solution of **Calendula Tincture** using ten drops of solution in a cup of warm water. Cover the wound and moisten with a few drops of the solution. It will help heal the wound promptly.

ABSCESSES

This refers to skin conditions where there is redness, pus, and infection of tissue.

When irritation is accompanied by redness and throbbing pain:
>Homeopathic Remedy: **Belladonna** (give every two hours, less frequently as improvement is evident)
>Bach Remedy: **Rescue Remedy** (placed on the abscess itself)
>Color Remedy: **Indigo**

Where there is pus and skin is sensitive to touch:
>Homeopathic Remedy: **Hepar Sulph** (every two hours until pus discharges or disappears)
>Bach Remedy: **Rescue Remedy**
>Color Remedy: **Violet**

When the skin is very tense and painful:
>Homeopathic Remedy: **Hypericum**
>Bach Remedy: **Rescue Remedy Cream** (on the abscess)

After discharge of pus, use three times a day for three days:
>Homeopathic Remedy: **Silica**
>Bach Remedy: **Rescue Remedy Cream** (topically)
>Color Remedy: **Indigo**

For mouth abscesses:
>Homeopathic Remedy: **Merc. Sol**
>Bach Remedy: **Rescue Remedy** (in water for gargling)
>Color Remedy: **Turquoise**

For general care, bathe affected part:

Homeopathic Remedy: **Calendula Lotion** (Put twenty drops of the tincture in a glass of hot water. Repeat three times daily to help the tissue open and heal.) All glandular abscesses should be seen by a physician.

ACCIDENTS

The first remedy to think of in any accident is **Arnica**. It is effective in easing shock; it also works as an anti-hemorrhagic to stop bleeding, and it will stop bruising of soft tissue, flesh, and muscle.

Homeopathic Remedy: **Arnica 30** (Needs to be given immediately after any accident and it can be repeated every fifteen minutes in serious conditions until medical help is available. If the accident is not serious, but shock or bruising are evident, give **Arnica 6** every half hour for 2–3 doses. Always remember that as symptoms disappear the remedy is needed less often. Other remedies can be administered, depending upon the type of injury. Please note any other symptoms that may accompany the accident. Check carefully for concussion, bleeding, and broken bones. Consult a physician if the condition of the patient is not better after first aid treatment.)

Bach Remedy: **Rescue Remedy** (Use for any accident, especially when the patient is in shock. This will help release shock from the system, and may need to be repeated every ten to fifteen minutes to bring peace of mind and relief from fear or anxiety.)

Color Remedy: **Spectrum** (restores energy depletion from an accident)

ACIDITY (STOMACH)

This can come on as a result of overeating, stressful conditions, fear, anxiety, or anticipation. Pay attention to the emotional state of the patient.

Acidity which may come on from being nervous about a future event such as exams, rehearsals, etc.:

Homeopathic Remedy: **Arg. Nit**

Bach Remedy: **Aspen**

Color Remedy: **Indigo**

Acidity accompanied by severe heartburn after small amounts of food, made worse from cold food and drink around four to eight P.M.:

Homeopathic Remedy: **Lycopodium**

Bach Remedy: **Cherry Plum**

Color Remedy: **Green**

ACNE

There are many types of acne. This is meant to cover general symptoms. If acne persists see a physician or consult a homeopath.

In people with red faces:

Homeopathic Remedy: **Belladonna**

Bach Remedy: **Pine**

Color Remedy: **Indigo**

With many pustules:

Homeopathic Remedy: **Hepar Sulph**

Bach Remedy: **Pine**

Color Remedy: **Indigo**

In people who have fair complexions:

Homeopathic Remedy: **Pulsatilla**

Bach Remedy: **Centaury**

Color Remedy: **Yellow**

When the skin becomes scarred from pustules:
 Homeopathic Remedy: **Silica**
 Bach Remedy: **Centaury**
 Color Remedy: **Violet/Magenta**
In cases that resist treatment of any nature:
 Homeopathic Remedy: **Sulphur**
 Bach Remedy: **Holly**
 Color Remedy: **Red**

APPENDICITIS

In any case where severe abdominal pain is present, a physician should be consulted immediately as complications can be very serious.

If a physician is not available:
 Homeopathic Remedy: **Iris Tenax** (Covers intense pain in the lower right side of the abdomen and tenderness to pressure in one area. Use 3x to 30x every two hours.)
 Bach Remedy: **Rescue Remedy** (Helps alleviate pain and discomfort until patient sees a physician.)
 Color Remedy: **Indigo**

APPETITE, EXCESSIVE

When there is a feeling of emptiness even after eating:
 Homeopathic Remedy: **Calc. Carb**
 Bach Remedy: **Gorse**
 Color Remedy: **Orange**
When the appetite is excessive and then goes to complete loss of appetite:
 Homeopathic Remedy: **Ferrum Phos.**
 Bach Remedy: **Mimulus**

Color Remedy: **Orange/Yellow**

Excessive appetite, even at night, and easily satisfied:

Homeopathic Remedy: **Lycopodium**

Bach Remedy: **White Chestnut**

Color Remedy: **Indigo**

APPETITE, LOSS OF

Aversion to all food, hunger stops person from sleeping:

Homeopathic Remedy: **Ignatia**

Bach Remedy: **Star of Bethlehem**

Color Remedy: **Spectrum**

A constant craving with a loss of appetite:

Homeopathic Remedy: **Arsen. Alb**

Bach Remedy: **Rock Water**

Color Remedy: **Orange**

APPREHENSION (ANXIETY)

There are many conditions and situations that can provoke apprehension. When these situations are stripping you of your vitality and energy these remedies can help considerably.

Anticipatory anxiety before an event such as an exam, a speech, or an important event which causes anxiety:

Homeopathic Remedy: **Arg. Nit** (Take a single dose of 30x the day before the event or a 6x a half hour before the event.)

Bach Remedy: **Aspen**

Color Remedy: **Green**

Apprehension accompanied with fear, diarrhea, trembling:

Homeopathic Remedy: **Gelsemium**

Bach Remedy: **Rescue Remedy**

Color Remedy: **Yellow**

ARTHRITIS

Homeopathic remedies are good for the relief of discomfort and pain associated with arthritis. For deeper treatment see a homeopath for constitutional treatment.

When the joints swell and are red and painful:

Homeopathic Remedy: **Apis Mel**

Bach Remedy: **Rescue Remedy Cream** (applied topically)

Color Remedy: **Violet**

When the joints feel bruised:

Homeopathic Remedy: **Arnica**

Bach Remedy: **Rescue Remedy Cream** (applied topically)

Color Remedy: **Violet**

When there appears to be no relief from pain:

Homeopathic Remedy: **Bryonia**

Bach Remedy: **Rescue Remedy tincture** (two drops in water, sip every half hour)

Color Remedy: **Magenta**

When pain shifts from joint to joint or extremity to extremity:

Homeopathic Remedy: **Pulsatilla**

Bach Remedy: **Wild Oat**

Color Remedy: **Indigo**

ASTHMA

Chronic asthma can be treated at a constitutional level by a homeopath. For acute attacks the following may stop symptoms and bring relief. Take a pill every fifteen minutes during an attack until there is improvement and then take less frequently or as needed.

When an attack is brought on by exertion or by speaking,

when there is tightness and pains in the chest, when breathing is oppressed and difficult:

Homeopathic Remedy: **Arnica**

Bach Remedy: **Rescue Remedy**

Color Remedy: **Green**

When an attack comes in the middle of the night with anxiety, restlessness, tossing, and inability to get comfortable in one position, burning heat in the chest, cold sweats and exhaustion that accompany the attack:

Homeopathic Remedy: **Arsen. Alb** (every ten minutes until attack diminishes, then less frequently)

Bach Remedy: **Rescue Remedy** (two drops in water, sipped every five minutes until nerves are steady and attack diminishes)

Color Remedy: **Turquoise**

When there is a tight, constricted feeling in the chest and rattling in the windpipe, which may feel full of mucus; when it is difficult to expectorate; when there is gasping for air, a pale face, cold feet, and sometimes nausea:

Homeopathic Remedy: **Ipecacuanha**

Bach Remedy: **Rescue Remedy** (two drops in water sipped at five minute intervals until patient shows marked improvement)

Color Remedy: **Green/Turquoise**

For "nervous asthma" where the person experiences suffocation, dizziness, coughing, vomiting, and nausea:

Homeopathic Remedy: **Lobelia Inflata**

Bach Remedy: **Rescue Remedy** (two drops in water, sipped every five minutes)

Color Remedy: **Green**

When an asthma attack, usually occurring in the early morn-

ing, is brought on by overeating and overdrinking, and the person feels very irritable:
    Homeopathic Remedy: **Nux Vom**
    Bach Remedy: **Rescue Remedy**
    Color Remedy: **Yellow**

BAD BREATH

When there is a bitter taste in the mouth on waking:
    Homeopathic Remedy: **Kali Phos**
    Bach Remedy: **Holly**
    Color Remedy: **Turquoise**
When there is a metallic taste in the mouth:
    Homeopathic Remedy: **Merc. Sol.**
    Bach Remedy: **Star of Bethlehem**
    Color Remedy: **Green**

BEREAVEMENT (GRIEF)

This may arise at any time one experiences loss. This can also be for losses felt acutely in the past that have not disappeared with time. Use for family members at a funeral or when a loved one is ill or in the hospital. It is better to allow the feelings to come to the surface than to suppress them.

When death comes very quickly and friends or family are in shock:
    Homeopathic Remedy: **Aconite**
    Bach Remedy: **Rescue Remedy**
    Color Remedy: **Magenta**
For grief that lingers:
    Homeopathic Remedy: **Ignatia**
    Bach Remedy: **Star of Bethlehem/Clematis**
    Color Remedy: **Magenta/Pink**

When grieving for an old rejection or loss:
　　Homeopathic Remedy: **Nat. Mur**
　　Bach Remedy: **Star of Bethlehem**
　　Color Remedy: **Magenta**

BITES, ANIMAL

These should be treated immediately by a physician.
Take immediately after the bite:
　　Homeopathic Remedy: **Aconite**
　　Bach Remedy: **Rescue Remedy**
　　Color Remedy: **Violet**

BLACK EYE

　　Homeopathic Remedy: **Arnica** (Give every hour for up
　　　　to five doses. If the bruising is relieved by cold cloths
　　　　use **Ledum** for five doses. If there is pain in the eyeball
　　　　use **Symphytum** every hour for three to four doses.)
　　Bach Remedy: **Rescue Remedy Tincture and Cream**
　　　　(applied locally to ease pain)
　　Color Remedy: **Indigo**

BLISTERS

　　Homeopathic Remedy: **Calendula Tincture** or **Oint-
　　　　ment** (Apply to the blister. If using tincture put ten
　　　　drops of solution into a small glass of hot water and
　　　　apply to the area. For internal use take **Causticum** 6x
　　　　morning and evening. Reduce intake as symptoms
　　　　disappear.)
　　Bach Remedy: **Rescue Remedy Cream** (applied topically
　　　　to soothe)
　　Color Remedy: **Indigo**

BOILS

When the skin is red, burning, and tight:
  Homeopathic Remedy: **Belladonna**
  Bach Remedy: **Beech/Rescue Remedy Cream** (applied
    topically)
  Color Remedy: **Indigo**
To cleanse the blood when a boil is festering:
  Homeopathic Remedy: **Gunpowder**
  Bach Remedy: **Holly/Rescue Remedy Cream** (applied
    topically)
  Color Remedy: **Yellow**
When an injury turns septic, and the boil is hot and painful:
  Homeopathic Remedy: **Hepar Sulph**
  Bach Remedy: **Rescue Remedy Cream** and **Tincture**
    (taken internally)
  Color Remedy: **Indigo**
When any injury festers and develops pus, and the boil is cold:
  Homepathic Remedy: **Silica**
  Bach Remedy: **Rescue Remedy Cream** and **Tincture**
    (taken internally)
  Color Remedy: **Green**
For very acute pain, inflammation, stinging, burning, and
throbbing, and the skin has gone to a purple color:
  Homepathic Remedy: **Tarantula Cubensis** (Externally
    bathe the boil in **Hypericum Tincture** using ten
    drops of tincture in warm water.)
  Bach Remedy: **Rescue Remedy Cream** and **tincture**
    (taken internally)
  Color Remedy: **Green**
As a preventative for recurring problems:
  Homeopathic Remedy: **Arnica**

BONES

For broken bones, to aid the healing process:
Homeopathic Remedy: **Symphytum**
Bach Remedy: **Aspen/Gentian**
Color Remedy: **Spectrum**
For fractured bones slow to mend:
Homeopathic Remedy: **Calc Phos**
Bach Remedy: **Gentian**
Color Remedy: **Spectrum**
Any bone injury mends well with:
Homeopathic Remedy: **Ruta Grav**
For bruised feeling in the bones:
Homeopathic Remedy: **Arnica**
If a bone injury was sustained and still aches:
Homeopathic Remedy: **Ruta Grav** (Use morning and night for a week. This can be repeated after a month if the treatment does not bring relief.)

BRONCHITIS

When there is rattling in the chest:
Homeopathic Remedy: **Ipecacuanha**
Bach Remedy: **Gorse/Rock Water**
Color Remedy: **Red**
When there is loss of voice or hoarseness:
Homeopathic Remedy: **Phosphorus**
Bach Remedy: **Olive**
Color Remedy: **Turquoise**
When accompanied by a fever and chills:
Homeopathic Remedy: **Arsen. Alb**
Bach Remedy: **Pine**
Color Remedy: **Orange**

With flu-like symptoms, bone ache, fever:
>Homeopathic Remedy: **Euphatorium**
>Bach Remedy: **Rescue Remedy** (sipped every half hour to relieve discomfort)
>Color Remedy: **Orange/Yellow**

BURNS

Serious burns should always be seen by a physician.

For shock:
>Homeopathic Remedy: **Arnica** (If accompanying fear give **Aconite** in place of **Arnica**.)
>Bach Remedy: **Rescue Remedy** (to calm nerves)
>Color Remedy: **Indigo**

To treat all burns:
>Homeopathic Remedy: **Cantharis**

When the pain of a burn is accompanied by restlessness and the skin blisters:
>Homeopathic Remedy: **Causticum** (Take a dose every half hour until the pain subsides.)

External application for burns:
>Homeopathic Remedy: **Urtica Urens Tincture** or **Hypericum Tincture** (In both remedies use ten drops in warm water and apply to the burn by dripping it over a sterile dressing. Do not remove the covering, but keep it moist at all times.)
>Bach Remedy: **Rescue Remedy Cream** (to ease pain and itching)

CARBUNCLES

If painful to the touch and patient finds contact from the dressing uncomfortable:

Homeopathic Remedy: **Hepar Sulph**
Bach Remedy: **Rescue Remedy Cream** (used topically)
Color Remedy: **Indigo**

To expel all pus and toxins:
Homeopathic Remedy: **Silica**
Bach Remedy: **Rescue Remedy Cream** (used topically)
Color Remedy: **Green/Yellow** (depending upon color of the pus)

If there is burning, stinging, and throbbing pain:
Homeopathic Remedy: **Tarantula Cubensis 6X**
Bach Remedy: **Rescue Remedy Cream** (used topically)
Color Remedy: **Violet**

When the skin is shiny and red, the pain is throbbing and stabbing, and when it is difficult to sleep:
Homeopathic Remedy: **Belladonna**
Bach Remedy: **Rescue Remedy Cream** (used topically)
Color Remedy: **Indigo**

For external treatment:
Homeopathic Remedy: **Hypericum Tincture** or **Cream**. (Follow treatment recommended for boils.)

CATARRH

For the treatment of chronic catarrhal conditions it is suggested you see a homeopath. Excess mucous conditions can be treated effectively.

When the patient has a head cold with thick yellow discharge:
Homeopathic Remedy: **Calc Fluor**
Bach Remedy: **Crab Apple**
Color Remedy: **Yellow**

With thick yellow discharge, weakness, and fretting:
Homeopathic Remedy: **Pulsatilla**

Bach Remedy: **Cerato**
Color Remedy: **Orange**
When there is stringy, glue-like discharge:
Homeopathic Remedy: **Kali Bich**
Bach Remedy: **Rescue Remedy**
Color Remedy: **Indigo**

CHEST PROBLEMS

Chest problems are often associated with flu-like symptoms.
With a dry painful cough:
Homeopathic Remedy: **Bryonia**
Bach Remedy: **Rescue Remedy**
Color Remedy: **Yellow**
With hoarseness and loss of voice:
Homeopathic Remedy: **Phosphorus**
Bach Remedy: **Rescue Remedy**
Color Remedy: **Turquoise**
When chest feels oppressed and person feels chilled:
Homeopathic Remedy: **Sulphur**
Bach Remedy: **Rescue Remedy**
Color Remedy: **Red/Orange**

CHILLINESS

When accompanied by desire to sit next to the fire or radiator:
Homeopathic Remedy: **Arsen. Alb**
Bach Remedy: **Rescue Remedy**
Color Remedy: **Orange**
With chronically cold hands:
Homeopathic Remedy: **Calc. Carb**
Bach Remedy: **Rescue Remedy**
Color Remedy: **Red**

When chilliness is intense with shivering:
Homeopathic Remedy: **Hepar Sulph**
Bach Remedy: **Rescue Remedy**
Color Remedy: **Red**
When chilly at night:
Homeopathic Remedy: **Sepia**
Bach Remedy: **Rescue Remedy**
Color Remedy: **Yellow**

COLDS

From sudden onset of symptoms (Often made worse after exposure to dry, cold winds. Patient feels fretful, even frightened, one cheek hot, the other cold.):
Homeopathic Remedy: **Aconite**
Bach Remedy: **Rescue Remedy** (two drops in water to be sipped to restore equilibrium)
Color Remedy: **Red**
When the symptoms are flu-like:
Homeopathic Remedy: **Gelsemium**
Bach Remedy: **Olive**
Color Remedy: **Spectrum**
When bones ache and flu has set in:
Homeopathic Remedy: **Euphatorium**
Bach Remedy: **Olive**
Color Remedy: **Spectrum**
Colds with much sneezing and running nose:
Homeopathic Remedy: **Nat. Mur**
Bach Remedy: **Rescue Remedy** (two drops in water to ease congestion and discomfort. Use cream on nostrils if they become irritated.)
Color Remedy: **Yellow**

COLIC

When there is gas, a distended belly like a drum, with tearing pains in the abdomen, gripping in the navel, and/or flatulent colic after anger, intolerance to pain, worse at night and in warmth:

Homeopathic Remedy: **Chamomilla**

Bach Remedy: **Rescue Remedy**

Color Remedy: **Yellow**

When the pains are made worse by eating and the belly is distended and there is relief in bending over:

Homeopathic Remedy: **Colchicum**

Bach Remedy: **Rescue Remedy**

Color Remedy: **Yellow**

When there are violent pains relieved by pressure and bending, the bowels feel as if they are being squeezed, and pain is acute:

Homeopathic Remedy: **Colocynthus**

Bach Remedy: **Rescue Remedy**

Color Remedy: **Yellow**

When pains abate from lying still and are better when not moving:

Homeopathic Remedy: **Bryonia**

Bach Remedy: **Rescue Remedy**

Color Remedy: **Violet**

When pains are better when doubled up:

Homeopathic Remedy: **Belladonna**

Bach Remedy: **Rescue Remedy**

Color Remedy: **Violet**

When pains are better with stretching, standing erect, and walking about, and/or flatulence is worse with pressure and doubling up:

Homeopathic Remedy: **Dioscorea**

Bach Remedy: **Rescue Remedy**

Color Remedy: **Green**

When pressure in the stomach feels like a stone; there is flatulence from eating "gassy" foods; frequent desire to move the bowels without effect; irritability; indicated for people who overeat and drink too much:

Homeopathic Remedy: **Nux Vom**

Bach Remedy: **Rescue Remedy**

Color Remedy: **Yellow**

For violent cramps radiating to all parts of the body; stomach feels as if it is drawn into the spine by a string; belly feels hard and bowels are constipated:

Homeopathic Remedy: **Plumbum**

Bach Remedy: **Rescue Remedy**

Color Remedy: **Violet**

For sharp pains as if cut by a knife; violent nausea and vomiting; guts feel as if they are tied in knots; sweating all over, very weak and sometimes passing out or in stupor:

Homeopathic Remedy: **Veratrum Alb**

Bach Remedy: **Rescue Remedy**

Color Remedy: **Yellow**

CONCUSSION

Always see a physician after a concussion.

When the trouble is not severe:

Homeopathic Remedy: **Arnica 30** (every fifteen minutes for four doses)

Bach Remedy: **Rescue Remedy**

Color Remedy: **Spectrum**

CONSTIPATION

For persistent constipation seek a homeopath. For acute bouts, which may come from time to time, look at one of the following remedies:

With ineffectual urging to move bowels:
Homeopathic Remedy: **Nux Vom**
Bach Remedy: **Water Violet**
Color Remedy: **Red**

When motions recede or feces are only partially expelled:
Homeopathic Remedy: **Silica**
Bach Remedy: **Wild Oat**
Color Remedy: **Yellow**

For large, painful motions:
Homeopathic Remedy: **Sulphur**
Bach Remedy: **Rescue Remedy**
Color Remedy: **Orange**

COUGHS

Croup-like cough, in spasms:
Homeopathic Remedy: **Calc Fluor**
Bach Remedy: **Rescue Remedy**
Color Remedy: **Green**

When croup-like cough comes after midnight:
Homeopathic Remedy: **Hepar Sulph**
Bach Remedy: **Rescue Remedy**
Color Remedy: **Green**

When croup-like cough is accompanied by fright:
Homeopathic Remedy: **Ignatia**
Bach Remedy: **Rescue Remedy**
Color Remedy: **Yellow**

Dry, painful coughing fits:
    Homeopathic Remedy: **Bryonia**
    Bach Remedy: **Rescue Remedy**
    Color Remedy: **Turquoise**
Sudden and violent coughing:
    Homeopathic Remedy: **Drosera**
    Bach Remedy: **Rescue Remedy**
    Color Remedy: **Yellow**
Persistent coughing, worse at night, particularly in children:
    Homeopathic Remedy: **Spongia**
    Bach Remedy: **Rescue Remedy**
    Color Remedy: **Turquoise**
With hoarseness, loss of voice, glassed-over eyes:
    Homeopathic Remedy: **Phosphorus**
    Bach Remedy: **Rescue Remedy**
    Color Remedy: **Turquoise**
Spasmodic fits of coughing, tightness in chest:
    Homeopathic Remedy: **Cuprum**
    Bach Remedy: **Rescue Remedy**
    Color Remedy: **Green**

CRAMPS

When cramps are in calf and are caused by exhaustion:
    Homeopathic Remedy: **Arnica**
    Bach Remedy: **Rescue Remedy**
    Color Remedy: **Red**
Cramps in calf muscles:
    Homeopathic Remedy: **Arsen. Alb**
    Bach Remedy: **Rescue Remedy**
    Color Remedy: **Red**

Cramps in legs and feet with contracted muscles, or for cramps in fingers and/or toes:

Homeopathic Remedy: **Cuprum**

Bach Remedy: **Rescue Remedy**

Color Remedy: **Red**

An effective remedy for any type of cramping:

Homeopathic Remedy: **Ledum**

Bach Remedy: **Rescue Remedy**

Color Remedy: **Red, Orange,** or **Pink**

When cramping starts at night, affects soles of the feet and person feels the need to stretch:

Homeopathic Remedy: **Nux Vom**

Bach Remedy: **Rescue Remedy**

Color Remedy: **Yellow**

When cramps occur only during the day and while sitting:

Homeopathic Remedy: **Rhus Tox**

Bach Remedy: **Rescue Remedy**

Color Remedy: **Orange**

CRUSHED FINGERS OR TOES

For body parts, such as fingers or toes, that have many nerve endings and are very sensitive:

Homeopathic Remedy: **Hypericum** 6x (taken internally every five minutes)

To alleviate symptoms of shock:

Homeopathic Remedy: **Arnica** (intermittently)

Bach Remedy: **Rescue Remedy** (to alleviate the emotional angst that accompanies injury)

Color Remedy: **Spectrum** (to bring balance back to the body); **indigo** (for pain)

CUTS

To stop bleeding:
Homeopathic Remedy: **Arnica** (can be repeated every
minute until bleeding ceases)
Bach Remedy: **Rescue Remedy**
Color Remedy: **Indigo**
For external application use:
Homeopathic Remedy: **Hypericum Cream** or **Tincture.**

CYSTITIS

When it is painful to urinate and there is a stinging feeling:
Homeopathic Remedy: **Apis Mel**
When the above symptoms occur and there is fever:
Homeopathic Remedy: **Belladonna**
When there is frequent urination and a burning feeling:
Homeopathic Remedy: **Cantharis**
When there are pink deposits in the urine:
Homeopathic Remedy: **Lycopodium**
When symptoms shift from place to place and patient is upset:
Homeopathic Remedy: **Pulsatilla**
Bach Remedy: **Rescue Remedy** (two drops in water,
sipped regularly to alleviate pain)
Color Remedy: **Indigo** (for pain)

DENTAL PROBLEMS

To alleviate dental shock and to control pain and bleeding:
Homeopathic Remedy: **Arnica**
Whenever there is nerve pain:
Homeopathic Remedy: **Hypericum**
When there is great fear of visiting the dentist:
Homeopathic Remedy: **Aconite**

When there is great sensitivity to pain, especially in young people:

Homeopathic Remedy: **Chamomilla**

For sharp darting pains following drilling:

Homeopathic Remedy: **Hypericum**

For excessive bleeding following drilling or tooth pulling:

Homeopathic Remedy: **Phosphorus**

For healing a pulled tooth:

Homeopathic Remedy: **Calendula Tincture** (as a mouthwash)

To strengthen weak and bleeding gums:

Homeopathic Remedy: **Fragaria Tincture** (as a mouthwash; ten drops in water)

Bach Remedy: **Rescue Remedy** (for pain and tension)

Color Remedy: **Turquoise** (for any teeth problems)

DIARRHEA

These remedies may be taken at hourly intervals for up to four doses. If diarrhea persists seek medical advice.

When there is a constant urging to motion but uncertainty whether gas or feces will pass, or after passing a movement the patient is exhausted and sweats profusely:

Homeopathic Remedy: **Aloe**

From food poisoning, excessive amounts of fruit, ice cream, or cold drinks in hot weather; nausea, vomiting, restlessness, heat, and burning sensations; patient is very weak and body parts are chilled:

Homeopathic Remedy: **Arsen. Alb**

For frequent, watery bowel movements with gas; painless, with undigested bits of food; weakness, delicacy, associated with summer diarrhea:

Homeopathic Remedy: **China**

For watery, yellow diarrhea after eating and drinking; pains are relieved by bending over:

Homepathic Remedy: **Colocynthus**

When diarrhea is caused by change of weather from hot to cold, or from getting wet; bowel movements are slimy green or yellow; loss of appetite and thirst:

Homeopathic Remedy: **Dulcamara**

When diarrhea is gushing, squirting, profuse, painless; cramps relieved by bending over and better with warm applications to belly; weak feeling persists:

Homeopathic Remedy: **Podophyllum**

When diarrhea is watery and profuse with cramps and colicky feeling; great thirst for ice water or acid drinks; violent nausea and vomiting; icy cold sweat:

Homeopathic Remedy: **Veratrum Alb**

When diarrhea comes on after antibiotics; smelly, offensive bowel movement; patient is irritable and exhausted after bowel movements:

Homeopathic Remedy: **Nitric Acid**

When diarrhea is offensive and drives patient out of bed in the morning:

Homeopathic Remedy: **Sulphur**

Bach Remedy: **Rescue Remedy** (two drops in water, sipped slowly helps alleviate pain, cramps, and fear)

Color Remedy: **Indigo**

DYSPEPSIA (HEARTBURN)

When the symptoms come from nervous anticipation of future events:

Homeopathic Remedy: **Arg. Nit**

When there is gas, patient craves fresh air, and is chilly
Homeopathic Remedy: **Carbo Veg**
When symptoms appear after small amounts of food, with pain, around four to eight P.M.:
Homeopathic Remedy: **Lycopodium**
When there is an acute sensation of burning:
Homeopathic Remedy: **Phosphorus**
Bach Remedy: **Rescue Remedy**
Color Remedy: **Indigo**

EARACHE

Avoid putting anything in the ear. When you select the appropriate remedy, give a dose hourly for up to three doses, and less frequently as symptoms disappear. As symptoms improve, give every two hours for a day and then three times daily for a day. If trouble persists see a physician.

When there has been exposure to cold air or wind and a fever, restlessness, and anxiety. Violent pain is better with warmth:
Homeopathic Remedy: **Aconite**
When pain develops suddenly and is severe; skin is dry and the face hot and red; the patient has no thirst and is restless:
Homeopathic Remedy: **Belladonna**
When the patient is very sensitive to pain, and it is worse with warm applications. A child is very cross and irritable. Sometimes in small children you notice one cheek is red and hot, the other white and cool:
Homeopathic Remedy: **Chamomilla**
When pain begins in the early stages and there is inflammation:
Homeopathic Remedy: **Ferrum Phos.**
When the patient is worse in drafts and sensitive to touch, wants to be warm and snug:

Homeopathic Remedy: **Hepar Sulph**

When the inflammation is in the inner ear:

Homeopathic Remedy: **Merc. Sol** (Give a dose every hour, then as pain eases off give every two hours until pain is gone.)

When there is throbbing and the ear feels stopped up. The patient wants air, is worse if it is warm in the evening, is very weepy, and in want of companionship and sympathy:

Homeopathic Remedy: **Pulsatilla**

Bach Remedy: **Rescue Remedy** (calms the nerves and eases pain)

Color Remedy: **Turquoise/Indigo** (for pain in the head)

EXHAUSTION

When exhaustion comes after physical exertion:

Homeopathic Remedy: **Arnica**

When exhaustion comes on after a sickness:

Homeopathic Remedy: **Arsen. Alb**

When exhaustion comes after mental effort, or any time you need to keep the blood sugar up for long periods of activity, such as long-distance driving, childbirth, studying for exams:

Homeopathic Remedy: **Kali Phos**

Bach Remedy: **Olive**

Color Remedy: **Spectrum** (Repeat every hour till energy is restored.)

EYES (INFLAMED, BURNING, WATERING, OR SWOLLEN)

When unable to bear bright light:

Homeopathic Remedy: **Euphrasia**

When eyelids are puffy and swollen:

Homeopathic Remedy: **Apis Mel**

Bach Remedy: **Rescue Remedy**
Color Remedy: **Indigo**

FAINTING

Select a remedy, give every ten minutes until the patient is recovered.

When there is fainting from emotional upset:
Homeopathic Remedy: **Ignatia**
When there is fainting from excitement:
Homeopathic Remedy: **Coffea**
When fainting comes from a hot, stuffy room:
Homeopathic Remedy: **Pulsatilla**
When fainting comes from pain:
Homeopathic Remedy: **Aconite** or **Chamomilla** (latter used in childbirth to relieve pain)
When fainting is caused by the sight of blood:
Homeopathic Remedy: **Nux Vom**
When fainting is caused by the loss of blood:
Homeopathic Remedy: **China** (If difficult to administer a pill, dissolve it in a small amount of water and wet the lips.)
Bach Remedy: **Rescue Remedy** (Take drops internally and also place on the pulse points at the neck, temples, and wrists.)
Color Remedy: **Orange**

FEAR

When fear comes on after a frightening experience:
Homeopathic Remedy: **Aconite**
When fear becomes terror (of crowds, death, or a bad experience):
Homeopathic Remedy: **Arsen. Alb**

When there is fear of thunder or darkness:
    Homeopathic Remedy: **Phosphorus**
When there is fear of appearing before groups of people:
    Homeopathic Remedy: **Arg. Nit**
When there is fear of failing at something (exams, interviews):
    Homeopathic Remedy: **Gelsemium**
    Bach Remedy: **Rock Rose/Mimulus**
    Color Remedy: **Yellow**

FOOD POISONING

When it is clear that sickness comes from spoiled food and the patient has diarrhea and is vomiting:
    Homeopathic Remedy: **Arsen. Alb**
When the poison comes from tainted fish:
    Homeopathic Remedy: **Carbo Veg**
    Bach Remedy: **Rescue Remedy**
    Color Remedy: **Yellow**

FRACTURES

Always see the appropriate medical staff to set the bones properly.
For shock:
    Homeopathic Remedy: **Arnica**
For pain and shock immediately following the accident:
    Bach Remedy: **Rescue Remedy**
An old-fashioned bone-healing remedy to ensure the bones knit properly:
    Homeopathic Remedy: **Symphytum** (three times daily for two weeks)
To ensure that bones are properly healed:
    Homeopathic Remedy: **Calc Phos** (may be given for a further four weeks)

Bach Remedy: **Rescue Remedy**
Color Remedy: **Spectrum**

GRIEF

Grief can be the etiology for many illnesses. It affects most people at some time in their life. Remedies can be used for personal loss and for situations where disturbing news of any kind sends a person into a state of grief or loss.

When there is silent brooding, sadness, hysteria, or deep crying:
Homeopathic Remedy: **Ignatia** (three times daily for a week)
When there is deep depression from grief and the patient shuns consolation and wishes to be alone with their grief:
Homeopathic Remedy: **Nat. Mur**
When grief turns to indolence, indifference, despair, or apathy:
Homeopathic Remedy: **Phos Ac.** (Give the same dose and for the same period of time as **Ignatia.**)
Bach Remedy: **Star of Bethlehem**
Color Remedy: **Magenta/Violet**

HAY FEVER

When eyes are burning and watery:
Homeopathic Remedy: **Euphrasia**
When all symptoms are better outdoors:
Homeopathic Remedy: **Pulsatilla**
In people prone to being chilly, sedentary, and weak:
Homeopathic Remedy: **Silica**
Bach Remedy: **Rescue Remedy**
Color Remedy: **Green**

HEADACHE

When you have selected the appropriate remedy for your type of headache, give a dose every ten minutes until symptoms are markedly reduced.

When there are sudden, violent pains with a burning sensation, as if the brain was in boiling water, the pain is intolerable, there is throbbing in the temples, the patient is restless, fearful, and thirsty:

Homeopathic Remedy: **Aconite**

When headaches reoccur periodically and the patient is weakened by them. Sometimes pain is relieved by vomiting. There is great thirst and the patient will take frequent sips of cool water. The patient is restless, fearful, and feels better when moving:

Homeopathic Remedy: **Arsen. Alb**

When there is sudden pain, throbbing, bursting sensation, the pain is worse with moving, bending, and moving the eyes. The head is hot, and the face flushed. The patient can't bear light or noise. Headache often begins in the afternoon and lasts throughout the night:

Homeopathic Remedy: **Belladonna** (These headaches can come after too much exposure to sun or heat, violent emotions, or periods.)

When a headache comes on from eating rich food or too much exertion and is accompanied by great thirst or no desire for movement of any kind, is worse on the left side, and patient lingers in bed:

Homeopathic Remedy: **Bryonia**

When a headache comes on with acute sickness or great anxiety, begins in the nape of the neck and settles over the eyes. It is often worse on the right side. The patient feels heavy, sleepy, and drowsy. Sometimes the person is shivery with chills, shows no thirst, and feels better after vomiting:

Homeopathic Remedy: **Gelsemium**

When pains are violent, pulsating, throbbing, or bursting, made worse by light and bending the head backwards. These headaches are always made worse by exposure to sun or heat. The patient will actually grab their head in pain. They are flushed and hot to the touch. They cannot bear to be touched and feel better in cold air and with cold applications:

Homeopathic Remedy: **Glonine**

When the headache feels like hammers inside the head, stitching pain in the head, a sore, bruised feeling around the eyes, and movement makes the headache worse. Headache starts in the back of the neck and spreads all over the head. It can be a blinding headache, often associated with PMS or mental exertion:

Homeopathic Remedy: **Nat. Mur**

When the headache is accompanied with vomiting and nausea caused by eating rich food and drink or excessive anger. Headache feels as if a nail is being driven into the head. The patient is worse with conversation, excitement, or movement, and is very irritable and chilly. Almost always constipated as well:

Homeopathic Remedy: **Nux Vom**

When the headache is in the temples and the head is hot, better with cold applications and fresh air. This is often associated with delayed or suppressed menstrual periods. The patient is dizzy when bending over and feels worse in a stuffy room or in areas with noise and light:

Homeopathic Remedy: **Pulsatilla**

Bach Remedy: **Rescue Remedy** (taken internally and a

compress of two drops of solution on a damp cloth
applied to head and neck)
Color Remedy: **Violet**

HEATSTROKE

When the pupils are dilated, there is a bounding pulse, burning, skin is hot and dry, patient has no thirst and is often delirious:
Homeopathic Remedy: **Belladonna**
When there is a painful headache with nausea and sometimes vomiting, and the patient is worse when moving:
Homeopathic Remedy: **Bryonia**
When there is a throbbing, bursting headache, flushed appearance, and the patient is sweating:
Homeopathic Remedy: **Glonine**
Bach Remedy: **Rescue Remedy** (taken internally and on a compress)
Color Remedy: **Indigo**

HOARSENESS

When the weather is cold and damp:
Homeopathic Remedy: **Carbo Veg**
With laryngitis:
Homeopathic Remedy: **Phosphorus**
Bach Remedy: **Rescue Remedy** (Gargle with water and two drops of solution.)
Color Remedy: **Turquoise**

HORSEFLY BITES

To bring the swelling down:
Homeopathic Remedy: **Hypericum**

Bach Remedy: **Rescue Remedy** (applied topically)
Color Remedy: **Indigo**

INDIGESTION

When accompanied with gas:
Homeopathic Remedy: **Carbo Veg**
From nervous tension:
Homeopathic Remedy: **Kali Phos**
From overeating or rich foods:
Homeopathic Remedy: **Nux Vom**
With headache and great thirst:
Homeopathic Remedy: **Bryonia**
Bach Remedy: **Rescue Remedy**
Color Remedy: **Yellow**

INSECT BITES

When there is numbness, sensitivity to being touched, and pain that is relieved by cold applications:
Homeopathic Remedy: **Ledum**
When there is burning, stinging pain made worse by the application of heat. There is swelling and the area is red and swollen:
Homeopathic Remedy: **Apis Mel**
When there is serious inflammation with burning, worse with touch but better with gentle massage:
Homeopathic Remedy: **Cantharis**
For insect bites:
Homeopathic Remedy: **Hypericum**
For insect stings:
Homeopathic Remedy: **Apis Mel** (Use **Arnica Tincture** or **Calendula Tincture** topically to relieve the stinging.)

Bach Remedy: **Rescue Remedy** (applied topically and
taken internally)
Color Remedy: **Violet/Indigo**

INSOMNIA

When there is twisting and turning and person cannot settle:
Homeopathic Remedy: **Aconite**
From being overly tired, the bed feels strange and hard:
Homeopathic Remedy: **Arnica**
When there are accompanying nightmares, jerking, screaming:
Homeopathic Remedy: **Belladonna**
Much yawning but unable to sleep:
Homeopathic Remedy: **Ignatia**
*When the feet and legs are hot and must be placed outside the
bed:*
Homeopathic Remedy: **Sulphur**
When the mind is full of ideas and can't be turned off:
Bach Remedy: **Rescue Remedy** (Sip from a glass of
water with 2 drops in it.)
Color Remedy: **Violet**

JOINTS

Swollen, painful:
Homeopathic Remedy: **Belladonna**
When there is rheumatism and pain:
Homeopathic Remedy: **Rhus Tox**
Bach Remedy: **Rescue Remedy**
Color Remedy: **Indigo**

MENSTRUAL PAINS

When the breasts are tender and swollen:

Homeopathic Remedy: **Calc. Carb**
When period is accompanied by headaches:
Homeopathic Remedy: **Calc Phos**
When depression accompanies the period:
Homeopathic Remedy: **Lycopodium**
When sad and irritable before and during period:
Homeopathic Remedy: **Nat. Mur**
When tearful with painful breasts:
Homeopathic Remedy: **Pulsatilla**
With cramps before and during period:
Homeopathic Remedy: **Mag. Mur**
Bach Remedy: **Rescue Remedy**
Color Remedy: **Orange/Magenta**

NAUSEA

Nausea with burning pains in the stomach and gut area:
Homeopathic Remedy: **Arsen. Alb**
Nausea and vomiting:
Homeopathic Remedy: **Ipecacuanha**
Nausea with vomiting after drinking alcohol:
Homeopathic Remedy: **Kali Bich**
Nausea and vomiting from smelling food:
Homeopathic Remedy: **Sepia**
Nausea with vomiting after eating rich food:
Homeopathic Remedy: **Nux Vom**
Bach Remedy: **Rescue Remedy**
Color Remedy: **Yellow**

NEURALGIA

When the pain disappears during the night and appears during the day:

Homeopathic Remedy: **Actaea Rac**
When the face is flushed, hot, and pain is throbbing:
Homeopathic Remedy: **Belladonna**
With severe pain:
Homeopathic Remedy: **Colocynthus**
Bach Remedy: **Rescue Remedy**
Color Remedy: **Violet**

NOSE

Nosebleeds in children:
Homeopathic Remedy: **Ferr. Phos.**
Frequent nosebleeds:
Homeopathic Remedy: **Hammamelis**
Nosebleeds caused from a blow:
Homeopathic Remedy: **Arnica**
Nosebleeds with profuse bleeding:
Homeopathic Remedy: **Phosphorus**
Nose running during colds and flu:
Homeopathic Remedy: **Gelsemium**
Nose running constantly without stopping:
Homeopathic Remedy: **Nat. Mur**
Bach Remedy: **Rescue Remedy**
Color Remedy: **Indigo**

SCIATICA

When discomfort is worse in cold, damp weather and at night:
Homeopathic Remedy: **Rhus Tox**
Bach Remedy: **Rescue Remedy** (Use cream in area
where sciatica is worse.)
Color Remedy: **Red**

SEASICKNESS

When there is nausea, dizziness, feeling of faintness, and loss of direction. When traveling by sea take one every hour and also a few minutes before departure:

Homeopathic Remedy: **Cocculus Indicus**

When there is nausea with saliva in the mouth, and/or vomiting and dizziness which is better when having food in the mouth:

Homeopathic Remedy: **Petroleum**

When the patient feels icy cold, has a sinking feeling in the stomach, and is worse with the smell of tobacco smoke:

Homeopathic Remedy: **Tobaccum**

Bach Remedy: **Rescue Remedy**

Color Remedy: **Yellow**

SHINGLES

When the scalp is affected:

Homeopathic Remedy: **Rhus Tox**

Bach Remedy: **Rescue Remedy**

Color Remedy: **Green**

SINUS DISORDERS

When there is excess mucus with stringy discharge:

Homeopathic Remedy: **Kali Bich**

When there is great pain in the face and head, sometimes with nausea:

Homeopathic Remedy: **Nat. Mur**

When the pain starts at the back of the head and settles over the face:

Homeopathic Remedy: **Silica**

Bach Remedy: **Heather/Larch**
Color Remedy: **Magenta**

SKIN

When the skin is blotchy:
Homeopathic Remedy: **Arg. Nit**
When the skin is cracked and there is weeping eczema:
Homeopathic Remedy: **Graphites**
When the skin feels better when scratching:
Homeopathic Remedy: **Calc. Carb**
When the skin itches and is worse when hot:
Homeopathic Remedy: **Merc. Sol**
When the skin itches and begins to burn:
Homeopathic Remedy: **Sulphur**
Bach Remedy: **Rescue Remedy Cream** (applied topically)
Color Remedy: **Indigo**

SPINE

When the nerve endings of the coccyx are injured:
Homeopathic Remedy: **Hypericum** (Give immediately
    and repeat night and day for three days or until pain
    subsides.)
When there is extensive bruising:
Homeopathic Remedy: **Arnica**
When the bone feels bruised:
Homeopathic Remedy: **Ruta Grav**
Bach Remedy: **Rescue Remedy**
Color Remedy: **Orange**

SPLINTERS

To expel the splinter:

Homeopathic Remedy: **Silica** (Three times daily for a few days. If it does not expel, see a physician.)

Apply to wounded area:

Homeopathic Remedy: **Calendula Tincture** (Put ten drops of tincture in a cup of hot water. If there is deep penetration of the skin give **Ledum** three times in four hourly intervals.)

Bach Remedy: **Rescue Remedy Cream**

Color Remedy: **Violet**

SPRAINS

When the sprain first occurs:

Homeopathic Remedy: **Arnica**

When the sprain continues to hurt:

Homeopathic Remedy: **Rhus Tox**

When the ligaments are affected:

Homeopathic Remedy: **Ruta Grav**

Bach Remedy: **Rescue Remedy**

Color Remedy: **Violet**

STIES

When there is a sticky discharge:

Homeopathic Remedy: **Graphites**

With a burning feeling in the eye:

Homeopathic Remedy: **Phosphorus**

At the beginning of the sty formation:

Homeopathic Remedy: **Pulsatilla**

If accompanied with a sore throat:

Homeopathic Remedy: **Nux Vom**

Bach Remedy: **Rescue Remedy** (taken internally and applied as a cream externally)

Color Remedy: **Indigo**

STOMACH PAINS

When there is burning in the stomach with a feeling of chill and sickness:
Homeopathic Remedy: **Arsen. Alb**
When food sits in the pit of the stomach like a stone:
Homeopathic Remedy: **Bryonia**
Bach Remedy: **Rescue Remedy**
Color Remedy: **Yellow**

SUNBURN

When the skin is red, hot, and throbbing, with no thirst:
Homeopathic Remedy: **Belladonna**
After a day in the sun when highly exposed to sun's rays:
Homeopathic Remedy: **Cantharis**
If sweating and cramping occur:
Homeopathic Remedy: **Cuprum**
Bach Remedy: **Rescue Remedy**
Color Remedy: **Indigo**

TEETHING IN BABIES

To give a remedy to a baby, you can dissolve the remedy in water or milk and either give in a bottle, or in small teaspoons as a dose. For nursing infants, the mother can take the remedy and pass the remedy on through nursing. Choose the appropriate remedy and give to the baby in fifteen-minute intervals until the baby is peaceful.

When the baby awakens in a fright, jerks, and jumps in their sleep; eyes are red, pupils dilated. They are hot to the touch, restless, and feverish; may even convulse and fall asleep instantly; gums are swollen and inflamed:

Homeopathic Remedy: **Belladonna**

When the baby's head is covered in sweat during sleep. They are fretful and irritable; feet may be cool and damp; bowel movements are light-colored. They vomit milk and have swollen bellies:

Homeopathic Remedy: **Calc. Carb**

When the baby is very irritable, crying, nothing will satisfy. They want to be carried all the time and will cry the minute they are put down to sleep. One cheek may be white, the other red:

Homeopathic Remedy: **Chamomilla**

When teething presents difficulties and the child is weak, delicate, and the teeth decay as soon as they appear:

Homeopathic Remedy: **Kreosotum**

Bach Remedy: **Rescue Remedy** (two drops in a bottle of water; let the baby sip at it)

Color Remedy: **Turquoise**

THIRST (EXCESSIVE)

When there is a high temperature:

Homeopathic Remedy: **Aconite**

When there is a craving for cold drinks:

Homeopathic Remedy: **Bryonia**

When there has been an excessive use of salt:

Homeopathic Remedy: **Nat. Mur**

When the mouth and throat are dry, craving milk:

Homeopathic Remedy: **Rhus Tox**

Bach Remedy: **Rescue Remedy**

Color Remedy: **Turquoise**

THIRST (LACK OF)

When the throat is swollen:
  Homeopathic Remedy: **Apis Mel**
When there is a high temperature:
  Homeopathic Remedy: **Gelsemium**
When the mouth is dry:
  Homeopathic Remedy: **Pulsatilla**
  Bach Remedy: **Rescue Remedy**
  Color Remedy: **Turquoise**

THROAT, SORE

When there has been exposure to cold winds:
  Homeopathic Remedy: **Aconite**
For immediate relief of pain:
  Homeopathic Remedy: **Kali Sulph** and **Nat. Phos**
    (Taken five minutes apart, repeat every half hour till
    symptoms disappear.)
When throat is sore, accompanied with constipation, irritability:
  Homeopathic Remedy: **Nux Vom**
When throat is painful and there is excessive saliva in the mouth:
  Homeopathic Remedy: **Merc. Sol**
  Bach Remedy: **Rescue Remedy** (to be sipped diluted in
    water)
  Color Remedy: **Turquoise**

TONSILLITIS

When there is inflammation and pain:
  Homeopathic Remedy: **Hepar Sulph**

Bach Remedy: **Rescue Remedy** (Gargle with water and two drops of solution.)

Color Remedy: **Turquoise**

TOOTHACHE

When there is an ache without any signs of inflammation or gumboils:
Homeopathic Remedy: **Kreosotum**
When there are no clear indications other than pain:
Homeopathic Remedy: **Merc. Sol**
When there is swelling, inflammation, and pain:
Homeopathic Remedy: **Apis Mel**
When the pain is made worse with cold drinks and air:
Homeopathic Remedy: **Calc. Carb**
When teeth are in poor condition:
Homeopathic Remedy: **Calc Fluor**
Bach Remedy: **Rescue Remedy** (two drops in water swished around the mouth)
Color Remedy: **Turquoise**

TRAVEL SICKNESS

When there is restlessness and fear:
Homeopathic Remedy: **Aconite**
When the least movement upsets:
Homeopathic Remedy: **Bryonia**
When there is irritability about movement and jarring:
Homeopathic Remedy: **Nux Vom**
When movement causes nausea and vomiting:
Homeopathic Remedy: **Ipecacuanha**
When symptoms of airsickness appear:

Homeopathic Remedy: **Belladonna**

Recovery from jet lag:

Homeopathic Remedy: **Arnica**

Bach Remedy: **Rescue Remedy** (every two hours)

Color Remedy: **Magenta**

VOMITING

When there is nausea, vomiting with faintness, sweating, and a disgust for food; vomiting of liquid as soon as it is taken; patient has no thirst:

Homeopathic Remedy: **Ant. Tart**

When there is vomiting of solid food and patient needs to keep still as the least movement makes the vomiting start again:

Homeopathic Remedy: **Bryonia**

When there is vomiting with constant nausea; vomiting empties stomach:

Homeopathic Remedy: **Ipecacuanha**

When there has been excessive overeating and drinking, vomits are sour smelling; the stomach is worse if any pressure is applied; the patient is irritable and chilled:

Homeopathic Remedy: **Nux Vom**

When vomiting is because of suppressed period or a chill on the stomach. Stomach craves rich, fatty food like mayonnaise, butter, pastry; craves cold water and cool air:

Homeopathic Remedy: **Pulsatilla**

Bach Remedy: **Rescue Remedy** (two drops of solution in water, sipped slowly)

Color Remedy: **Yellow**

WOUNDS

To clean out wounds immediately:

Homeopathic Remedy: **Calendula Tincture**

For puncture wounds:

Homeopathic Remedy: **Calendula and Ledum** (Take internally every hour for five doses, three doses the next day. If any sign of infection occurs see a physician.)

Bach Remedy: **Rescue Remedy**

Color Remedy: **Orange**

First Aid Materia Medica

ACONITE (ACONITUM NAPELLUS)

Aconite is advised for the sudden onset of all symptoms that usually come on after exposure to drafts, cold wind, or icy cold weather. The symptoms appear as a dry, suffocating cough, sore throat resulting from exposure to cold, dry wind and weather. A high temperature with a great thirst and all signs of illness appear very quickly. There can be acute pain which the patient finds intolerable.

It is also good for where fear is felt. Fear is another symptom that responds to *Aconite*: fear of crowds, death, approaching events, and/or the past. The person is always anxious, fretful, and is physically and mentally restless.

Symptoms can come on from bereavement, bites, travel, or anxiety. They are always worse at midnight, while lying on affected side, in a warm room, in cold air, in tobacco smoke, or while listening to music. They are relieved in airy rooms, or when the bedding is thrown off. Use *Aconite* at the beginning of a cold, sore throat, or the flu. It can stop these illnesses if you give it immediately when symptoms appear. This remedy does not have a long-term effect and is mainly for the beginning of illness. Use for shock and injury if there is fear.

The difference between *Aconite* and *Arnica* is that *Aconite* is for fear and *Arnica* is not.

ACTAEA RAC (ACTAEA RACEMOSA)

This remedy is for headaches and neuralgia, stiff necks and painful muscles following rigorous exercise. There is often rheumatism in the back and shooting pains along the spine. The patient who needs this remedy is confused, depressed, and despondent. They are worse in cold, damp weather and while moving. They are better in warmth or when eating; their headaches get better when they are outdoors.

ALOE

This is an excellent remedy when people have used a lot of drugs. It works for stagnant digestion, when people live a sedentary life. The psychological picture is suited for people who are dissatisfied and angry at themselves. They are hot, internally and externally. The belly feels full, heavy, and bloated. Their bowels feel loose and their limbs feel lame. They are worse in the morning, summer, heat, in hot, dry weather, and after eating and drinking. They feel better in cold, open air. The patient can have headaches alternating with lumbago and intestinal and uterine problems. There is a disinclination to mental work. The pure juice of *aloe* in homeopathic potency is good for consumption and digestive problems.

ANT. TART (ANTIMONIUM TARTARTICUM)

This remedy is used for rattling mucus in the chest made worse by the slightest expectoration. There is a sensation of great fatigue, weakness, and cold sweat. They are worse in the evening, lying down at night, and from warmth. They are better sitting erect, and after burping and expectoration. This is an excellent remedy for children with colds in their lungs and bronchia. The rattling noise is apparent to anyone near the patient and is the keynote symptom that calls for this remedy.

APIS MEL (APIS MELLIFICA)

This remedy is used for all the effects of insect stings and for symptoms where there is swelling, soreness, and intolerance to heat. The skin has a red, rosy hue. It is a remedy used for edema, congestion, and heat in any part of the body. There is always a burning, stinging sensation, whether it is with the symptoms of swollen eyes, or the burning sensation of cystitis. There is generally an absence of thirst. *Apis Mel* can be effective in the treatment of arthritis where joints are swollen and there is redness and burning. It is indicated where there is great irritability and depression resulting from anger, fright, and grief. Some of the symptoms that respond to this remedy are rheumatism, swollen parts, incontinence, and rash. Patients are often listless, have trouble concentrating, and can be despondent about their lives. They are worse during the late afternoon, after sleep, from heat, when touched, and in closed, heated rooms. They are better in the open air and with cold water.

ARG. NIT (ARGENTUM NITRICUM)

This remedy works on the throat, when the mucous membranes are affected and irritated. It is also an excellent remedy for nerves, irritable stomach symptoms, and suits fearful and nervous people. It is also used when the mind is full of anxieties and fear, the memory weak, and there are errors of perception.

It is a good remedy for mental exertion. It is also excellent for anticipation, when time appears to pass too slowly, stage fright, and examination nerves, or if one cannot stand heat and is worse in any form of warmth, at night, after eating, or has sweats. They are better in fresh air, when cold, and when burping. It is a good remedy when people are stressed from work and have long chronic periods of anxiety.

ARNICA

This is the first remedy to be thought of for shock, trauma, accident, or injury. It takes away the shock, which is always present in accidents. It is excellent for bruising and also acts as an anti-hemorrhagic. It will stop bleeding instantly and should be thought of in all wounds where there is bleeding and contusion to tissue. It relieves sore, bruised feelings after injury, and childbirth. If they say they want to be left alone and always tell you that they are all right, no matter how ill or shocked they may be, *Arnica* is the premiere homeopathic remedy. It is known to restore vitality after jet lag, and to stop bleeding, bruising, and soreness. Consider it first for any accident, injury, or shock. If you wish to apply it topically to a wound, never put it on cut skin. It will sting and cause irritation. Use it on bruised areas or where there is soreness and aching. It is excellent for any ache or pain. Use it before and after dentistry, before and after exertion, such as workouts, long cycling trips, or running. It will save wear and tear on the body and help your metabolism respond in ways that lead to prompt regeneration.

ARSEN. ALB (ARSENICUM ALBUM)

This remedy should be thought of whenever there is weakness, debility, exhaustion, and restlessness, with nightly aggravation around midnight to 2 A.M. It can revive a person during and after flu or serious illness, or with burning symptoms, and with unquenchable thirst, where the person sips drinks slowly. It is excellent for food poisoning and will bring equilibrium to the digestive system promptly. It is used with septic infections and low vitality after illness. When the patient needs this remedy, you will generally see such a restlessness around midnight that it can drive the patient from room to room. Think of this remedy for midnight to 2 A.M. asthma attacks. The patient may feel chilly, fastidious, and exacting. They are worse in cold air, with cold applications, at night, and between midnight and 2 A.M. They are better with warmth, except with a headache, and then they ask for cold applications. You may see the patient sitting wrapped in blankets by an open window. It is good for influenza, colds, and times of serious illness when pain and medication have exhausted the patient.

BELLADONNA

This remedy acts on the entire nervous system where there is congestion, inflammation, convulsions, and pain. It is always associated with hot, red skin, flushed face, glaring eyes, throbbing veins, and a state of excitation, violence, and anger. The sleep is restless; there can be delirium and pains that come and go suddenly and violently. This remedy works on a dry, parched throat where the patient does not wish to drink. Lack of thirst is a keynote symptom. It is a wonderful children's remedy and can stop a fever promptly. The patient is worse after 3 P.M. or after midnight, from uncovering or being in drafts, or lying down. They are better when their body is covered and their head held high. Think of this remedy for arthritic pains, fevers, and sore throats where there is sudden pain and inflammation. It can be used for throbbing, bursting headaches where patient is sensitive to light, and pain is worse on the right side, and when lying down. Remember that *Belladonna* cases are not thirsty and are hot. These are considered classic symptoms for the remedy.

BRYONIA

This remedy is for a person who suffers from or dislikes movement of any kind from headaches, mastitis, colds, and flu. The patient cannot stand to get out of bed. Movement makes all symptoms worse. The patient is irritated or angered. They are thirsty and crave cold water. They are anxious about the future and often insecure, which can produce headaches, or an illness symptomatic of not having to move forward in life. They prefer to stay where they are. Even food sits in the stomach and does not move, as if a stone were in the pit of the stomach. There is often accompanying constipation. This remedy should be thought of for headaches (worse on the left side), colds and coughs, hacking and dry. It is good for fevers where the patient is sweating and chilled. The patient is worse with movement, worse in the morning, from eating, from hot weather, exertion, and touch. They feel better lying on the painful part of the body, better with pressure, rest, and cold applications. Always think of *Bryonia* for migraine. For the treatment of chronic migraine consult a homeopath.

CALC. CARB (CALCAREA CARBONICA)

This remedy is good for over 90 percent of all children at some point in their homeopathic constitutional treatment. It is often thought of for patients who are fat, flabby, and obese. It affects nutrition, glands, skin, and bone. It is used for swellings, tickling coughs, fleeting chest pains, nausea, acidity, and a dislike of fat. The patient becomes out of breath easily. It is used when there are relapses, especially during colds with heavy mucus. The mental symptom is apprehension, which is worse toward evening. The patient is full of fears, is irrational, or fears that others will see their weakness. They can be confused, low-spirited, and forgetful. They can be obstinate and adverse to work and exertion. They may be overweight, have excessive appetites, dislike dairy products, and have a tendency to feel cold and catch cold easily. They may have itching skin and profuse periods. This remedy is suited to quiet, shy, sensitive people who are subject to depression, who are worse in cold, damp weather, and when standing. They are better in dry weather, from warmth and from lying on the painful side.

CALC FLUOR (CALCAREA FLUORICA)

This remedy is used when there is a thick, greenish discharge, excessive coughing and catarrh with tiny lumps. It is used in croup, for gumboils, toothache, and arthritis. The person is worse after rest, and from damp weather, and is better after a little movement and with warm applications.

CALC PHOS (CALCAREA PHOSPHORICA)

This remedy is excellent for broken bones that are slow to knit. It is good for slow dentition in children, anemic children who are peevish, have weak digestion, and are cold to the touch. This remedy is used for headaches after weather change, severe stomach pain after eating, and for heartburn. It is useful for period pains, acne, and inflamed gums. It is helpful after grief and after injury, and for those who are worse with any change in weather, especially cold, damp, rainy weather, and from exertion and movement. They are better in warm, dry weather, with hot baths, and when resting.

CALENDULA

This is the best remedy for cuts, incised wounds, and when there is injury to skin tissue in any form. It is applied topically to injuries to stop bleeding and to clean damaged tissue. It promotes quick and efficient healing to all tissue. It is suggested for cradle cap, cuts, wounds, incisions, and especially after surgery. Put ten drops of the tincture into a cup of hot water and apply to the area. Moisten bandaged wounds such as burns by dripping the solution over the wound. It can be used on eczema, rashes, and areas of the skin that are irritated. It brings soothing relief. The tincture can be applied in creams and used whenever there is irritation.

CANTHARIS VESICATORIA

This remedy is specific for all burns or burning pains. It is used for burns and scalds before blisters form; sunburn; burning in the bladder before, during, and after urination; in cystitis, when the urine scalds the skin; burning in the eyes, mouth, throat, and stomach. Burning is the keynote symptom made worse by touch, during urination, and after drinking cold water and coffee. The person feels better in warmth and when lying down. It will relieve the pain associated with all burning symptoms.

CARBO VEG (CARBO VEGETABILIS)

This is a wonderful remedy to help people revive after they have been ill and are weak. There may be anemia and depletion of all energy. It will revive people when they have fainted, and can be useful for coma and unconsciousness. It also offers temporary relief from belching, acidity, and gas in the intestines. It is a specific remedy after food poisoning from eating contaminated fish. It is good for ailments following cold, damp weather when the person may shiver but cling to an open window for fresh air. This remedy can be used for hoarseness and voice loss. Use it also with discomfort after eating fatty food, during warm, damp weather, and in the evenings and at night. It is good for belching and passing wind.

CAUSTICUM

This remedy is used for burning, and for rawness and soreness in parts of the body, such as the throat, chest, and rectum. There may be weakness, sinking strength, and shaking in the patient who needs this remedy. It is used often for incontinence when the patient coughs, sneezes, or blows their nose, or while walking or during sleep. It is for those who are worse in dry, cold winds, in fine weather, and in cold air, and are better in damp weather, warmth, or the heat of bed. This remedy is for patients broken down from a long disease, or extended worry. Sometimes paralysis is setting in and this can reverse the symptoms.

CHAMOMILLA

This is an excellent remedy for small children, especially during teething. It is used when children are peevish, restless, and angry, with an acute sensitivity to pain and changes. They may be irritable, thirsty, hot, and their pain seems unendurable. A child may whine, be given many things and reject them all. One cheek will be red and hot, the other white and cold. This strange, rare, and peculiar symptom is always an indication for this remedy. The remedy is used for toothache and excruciating pains, such as backache, childbirth, and rheumatic pains. It is made worse by heat, anger, open air, wind, and at night. The child feels better being carried, in warmth, and in wet weather.

CHINA

This is a remedy used for weariness and prostration. It is used as a general tonic and is especially good after malaria and asthma attacks, which occur periodically with weakness and exhaustion. It is good for fever accompanied by continuous weakness and depletion.

COCCULUS INDICUS

This is one of the great remedies for motion sickness with sensations of weakness or hollowness. The person suffers from lack of sleep or overwork. The head feels so heavy it can't support itself. In seasickness the patient is better in fresh air. They are worse after eating, from loss of sleep, in open air, with smoking, from riding, and in noise. It can be used in pregnancy with morning sickness and backache.

COFFEA

This remedy is used for pain relief for the patient who is nervous, sensitive, and excitable. It is used as a painkiller in childbirth and extreme pain due to injury or wounding, where the patient's nerves feel on edge. They feel worse with excessive emotions, joy, narcotics, strong odors, noise, in open air, cold, and at night. They are better in warmth, lying down, and sucking on ice.

COLOCYNTHUS

This is a wonderful remedy for the treatment of painful neuralgia. *Colocynthus* is suited for angry, irritable people. When pains are so severe that the person doubles over for relief, and all pains are relieved by bending forward, doubling up, hard pressure, warmth, and lying with head bent forward.

CUPRUM

This remedy is considered whenever spasms and cramps affect the body. These can be leg cramps, congestion and spasms in the lungs with asthma, or stomach cramps. *Cuprum* can be used for convulsions, violent contractions, and intermittent, spasmodic pain. Spasms begin with a twitching in the fingers and moving out. The patient is made worse from vomiting and nausea. They feel better perspiring and drinking cold water.

DIOSCOREA

This remedy is thought of primarily for colic in the belly, radiating out from the navel to all parts. The pain feels worse bending and is relieved by standing erect. Infants with colic try to stretch themselves fully to alleviate their discomfort. There may be wind and rumbling associated with stomach conditions. The patient feels worse lying down or doubled up, and is worse at night. They are better standing, stretching, in open air, and with pressure.

DROSERA

This is a remedy used specifically for spasmodic coughs. Any cough which is violent, protracted, and ends in vomiting responds to *Drosera*. Symptoms are deep, hoarse, barking coughs, constant tickling coughs, laryngitis with a dry throat that makes it difficult to speak, and a sensation of a feather in the back of the throat. The patient is worse with warmth, warm drinks, while laughing, singing, talking, when lying down, after midnight, and better in open air, with activity, and getting out of bed.

DULCAMARA

This remedy is used for symptoms caused by changes in

weather, especially from warm to cold. The person has stiffness in the joints, especially the back, neck, and throat. They suffer from diarrhea after exposure to wet weather conditions. They may also have rheumatic pains brought on by weather changes that are worse at night and in cold, damp, rainy weather. They feel better when warm and moving about.

EUPHATORIUM

This is one of the best remedies for flu when the bones ache, and there is a high fever and head congestion. It can take all the aches out of a bad bout of malaria or influenza, and is excellent for the aches and pains associated with any illness.

EUPHRASIA

This is specifically known as a remedy to treat inflammation of the eye, the conjunctiva, and when there is profuse tearing. The patient is better in open air. It is used when there is running of the eyes and nose often associated with hay fever and other irritants. It works to alleviate bursting headaches with dazzling eyes. The patient is worse indoors, in the evening, in warmth, and light. The patient feels better in the dark.

FERRUM PHOS. (FERRUM PHOSPHORICUM)

This remedy is best used to stop a fever in its early stages. It can also be used to stop a cold that is developing. It stops hemorrhages, especially nosebleeds. It will alleviate a frontal headache that is relieved by nosebleed. The person is worse at night between 4 and 6 A.M., and with touch and movement. The right side is worse. They feel better with cold applications.

FRAGARIA

This is a tincture made from wild strawberries that strengthens the gums and freshens the mouth.

GELSEMIUM

This is an excellent flu remedy where the patient is weak, trembling, and chilly. The eyes can barely stay open, there is a dull, tired headache, and the mind is dull. The patient is unable to think clearly. It relieves sore throats, symptoms of flushing, aching, and "tight" headaches. There may be an absence of thirst even with high fever and difficulty in swallowing. It is also an excellent remedy for anticipatory anxiety, such as rehearsals, school exams, and interviews. It takes the "stage fright" away. The patient is worse at 10 A.M., in hot rooms, exposed to the sun, and on receiving bad news. They feel better in the open air and after urinating.

GLONINE

This is used for bursting headaches that start in the back of the neck and are so painful that it feels like the head will explode. The patient cannot bear anything on their head and symptoms may be brought on by sunstroke or overheating. They are worse in the sun, with exposure to gas, open fire, stimulants, or when lying down or putting the head down. They are worse between 6 A.M. and 12 P.M.

GRAPHITES

This is used to treat unhealthy skin conditions, such as eczema, cracked fingers, or when there is a tendency for skin to suppurate. The patient is often overweight and constipated.

GUNPOWDER

This is used specifically as a blood cleaner for boils and carbuncles.

HAMMAMELIS

This is used as first aid for nosebleeds, tired feeling in arms and legs, burns, bruises, and whenever the mucous membranes are inflamed.

HEPAR SULPH (HEPAR SULPHURIS)

This remedy is used when injuries suppurate and weep, as with eczema, acne, and cracks in the lower lip. It is a wonderful remedy for croup, coughs brought on by exposure, wheezing, earaches, and tonsillitis. The patient feels worse in cold air, lying on the painful part, or when the affected part is touched. They feel better in warmth, and wrapped up in damp, cold weather.

HYPERICUM

This is an excellent remedy for healing lacerated wounds that involve areas of nerve endings—fingers, toes, and the coccyx. It is good for bites, abscesses, and any painful, deep wound to the body; it will promote healing rapidly. It can be used in a cream, tincture, or taken internally. The person is worse when it is cold and damp, when touched, or in a closed room. They are better bending the head backwards.

IGNATIA

This is considered the first remedy for grief, when tears are shed, and when the patient wants only to be left alone. It relieves fright, prolonged grief, and helps sore throats, croup, and backaches brought on by the structure breaking down in one's life. It helps insomnia where there is much yawning but no sleep. The patient is worse with tobacco, cold air, strong odors, and alcohol, and is better in warmth, when changing positions, and when eating.

IPECACUANHA

Any time there is nausea or vomiting this remedy relieves. It is good for travel sickness, morning sickness, and asthma with nausea. It relieves rattling mucus in the bronchial area when there is nausea and vomiting. The person is worse in winter and dry weather, as well as in a warm room where they can't get enough air. They are better with open air, resting with eyes closed.

IRIS TENAX

This remedy is specific for appendicitis and for headaches with vomiting.

KALI BICH (KALI BICHROMICUM)

This is a remedy for catarrhal conditions: sinus troubles, sore throats, and coughs with copious mucus. It is also for migraines, blurred vision, nausea, and vomiting after alcohol use. The patient is worse in the morning, when drinking, especially beer, and in hot weather. They are better with hot applications.

KALI PHOS (KALI PHOSPHORICUM)

This remedy is reserved for extreme exhaustion, when people are tired from overwork, nervous exhaustion, and from long periods of preparation for a project at school or work. It is used in stages of childbirth to keep the blood sugar up so that the mother can focus on delivering the baby. It is good for headaches with humming in the ears following long mental effort. The patient is worse with noise, excitement, and mental and physical exhaustion. They are better with nourishment, and light easy movement.

LEDUM

This is a remedy used for all puncture wounds from nails, pins, and needles, especially when there is little or no bleeding. It is to be used for bites from animals, such as horses, dogs, cats, and rats. If shooting pains develop after the bite or wound use *Hypericum*. This remedy can help avoid tetanus. *Ledum* can be used in varicose ulcers that refuse to heal. The patient is worse at night, from the heat of the bed, and better in cold, when uncovered, and using cold water, especially putting their feet in cold water.

LOBELIA INFLATA

This remedy is used specifically for asthma attacks, when the chest feels heavy and there is nausea and vomiting. The patient is worse in motion, cold, in the afternoon, and around tobacco. They are better in warmth, and at night.

LYCOPODIUM

This is a remedy that affects digestion and is good for acidity, hiccups, gout, and cystitis. It is used for excessive hunger, a preference to be alone, a dislike of exercise, when irritable, or when one craves sweets even though they cause indigestion. The patient is worse between 4 and 8 P.M., in stuffy rooms, in cold air, with food and liquid. They are sensitive to loud noise, and feel better with warm food and drinks, wearing loose clothes, in fresh air, and with activity.

MAG. MUR (MAGNESIA MURIATICUM)

This is used as first aid for menstrual cramping, often when there is acne preceding the menses, and flooding during the period. The person feels worse immediately after eating, lying on the right side, and bathing in the sea. They feel better with pressure, motion, and in open air.

MAGNESIA PHOSPHORICUM

This is used as an antispasmodic remedy. It is exceptionally good for muscle cramps of any nature. It is an asthma remedy, useful in dry, tickling coughs, spasmodic coughs, and whooping cough. The patient feels worse on the right side, from cold, touch, or at night. They are better in warmth, bending double, with pressure and friction.

MERC. SOL (MERCURIUS SOL)

This is suggested for feverish head colds with great weakness and shaking, for sore throats with overabundant saliva, mouth ulcers, thrush of the mouth, toothache, and earache. It is an excellent remedy for abscesses, and itching skin conditions. It is used if one has offensive breath, spongy, bleeding gums, or profuse, fetid sweats with no relief. The person is worse at night, in wet, damp weather, lying on their right side, and perspiring. They are better in a warm room and in a warm bed.

NAT. MUR (NATURM MURIATICUM)

This is the best remedy for running noses and sinus problems. It is useful in the treatment of eczema, urticaria, and with menstrual pains when the patient is sad, irritable, and has reoccurring PMS. It is suited for people who tend to feel insecure and unsure of themselves, who worry about the future, are easily moved to tears or unable to cry at all, or are very irritable before their periods. It is used for the ill effects of prolonged grief, fright, or anger, or if they want to be left alone to experience their sadness, or feel that they will never have a good life. The person is worse in noise, with music, in a warm room, about 10 A.M., at the sea, with mental exertion, consolation, and talking. They feel better in the open air, on bright, sunny days, and washing in cold water after a sweat.

NITRIC ACID

This is used for strong, splinter-like pains, or sticking pains. It is excellent for treating blisters and ulcers in the mouth, tongue, and genitals with discharges that are very offensive, or for people with chronic diseases who take cold easily and are disposed to diarrhea. It is effective when the mind is irritable, hateful, vindictive, hopeless, and in despair. The person may be sensitive to noise, touch, jarring, and often fears death. They are worse in the evening, at night, in cold climates, and in very hot weather. They feel better when driving.

NUX VOM (NUX VOMICA)

This remedy can cure a multitude of modern-day problems for people stuck in offices, who do not move a lot, and eat rich food and drink regularly. The patient may be very irritable, and sensitive to all impressions. They can be violent-tempered, even malicious. They are oversensitive to odor, noise, and light, and they do not want to be touched. *Nux Vomica* is used for hangovers, indulgence in rich food, and excessive drinking. It is a good nerve remedy, especially suited for travel sickness and indigestion. This is an excellent headache remedy, one used specifically for constipation, itching hemorrhoids, stuffy colds, raw sore throats, and PMS. The patient is worse in the morning, from mental exertion, after eating and using all stimulants and narcotics, and in cold weather. They feel better with sleep, damp, wet weather, and with strong pressure.

PETROLEUM

This is used for many skin conditions and for asthma attacks. It is used when tissue is irritated by external stimuli. *Petroleum* is good for lingering gastric and lung problems and chronic diarrhea. It is suitable for lasting complaints, fright, irritability, and fears of death. The patient is worse in dampness, before and during thunderstorms, in cars, and during winter. They are better in warm air and dry weather.

PHOS. AC (PHOSPHORIC ACID)

This is used when a patient is exhausted, weak, and nervous. It revives mental tiredness and physical exhaustion. It is useful after serious illnesses when people cannot regenerate their vitality. It is good for excesses, grief, and loss of fluids. It is also used to treat cancer pain.

PHOSPHORUS

This is an excellent remedy for bronchitis and chest problems. It helps cure coughs, hoarseness, laryngitis, and loss of voice. It also works on stomach symptoms, such as vomiting and heartburn. The patient craves cold water, but often vomits it back up when it becomes warm in the stomach. They fear thunderstorms and lightning. The patient is also very sensitive to noise, light, and the slightest stimulation. *Phosphorus* can be used after anesthesia to clear the system of ill effects, and is considered an excellent jet lag remedy. The patient is worse with touch, exertion, at twilight, with warm food and drink, changes of weather, from getting wet in hot weather, in thunderstorms, and ascending stairs. They feel better in the dark, eating cold food and drink, in the cold, open air, and having sleep.

PLUMBUM

This is good for treating weakness and paralysis in the limbs, or in conditions where there is progressive paralysis. The patient may be worse at night, and with motion. They may feel better with rubbing, hard pressure, and exertion.

PULSATILLA

This is known as the weather cock remedy because pains and symptoms are always shifting to one side or the other, or from one area of the body to another. *Pulsatilla* is thought of for shy, clinging children, people who crave fresh air and always feel better outdoors, even though they may be chilly. It is used when the mucous membranes are affected, secreting copious thick yellow-green discharges. The symptoms are always changing and the patient is complaining, whining, chilly, and is not thirsty.

The emotional state is that a patient weeps easily over trifles, is timid, fears being alone, and wants consolation from others. The patient is worse in heat, after rich food, after eating, in the evening, and in warm and stuffy rooms. They are better in open air, having windows open, even in winter, after cold food and drinks, and with motion.

RHUS TOX (RHUS TOXICODERNDRON)

This is a wonderful remedy for sprains and muscle strain. It can relieve rheumatism, lumbago, stiff neck, and pains made worse by proximity to dampness, moisture, and cold. When a person has been sitting or lying in one position for too long and the body becomes stiff and achy, this remedy brings swift relief. The person is worse with sleep, in cold, wet, damp, rainy weather, after rain or cold bathing, with night rest, and has right-sided complaints. They are better in warm, dry weather, in motion, walking, changing positions, with rubbing, using warm applications, and from stretching out the limbs.

RUTA GRAV

This remedy is for bruised bones, even old injuries where there is stiffness and bone pain. It works well where there is trouble with the wrists, and with conditions that are worse in cold, wet weather and when the person always feels better moving. It relieves eyestrain for close-up work, or when the eyes are weary and ache. The patient is worse lying down and when they are cold. It is useful for sprains, muscle strain, pulled ligaments, and backache.

SEPIA

This is a predominantly female remedy, used for period pains, nausea during pregnancy, and menopause that has many symptoms. The person is sensitive to cold, sad, and fearful of being left alone, and is emotionally indifferent to those close. *Sepia* is suited for people who are depressed, and who are fearful. The person is worse in the afternoons and evenings, from cold, thunder, and from tobacco smoke. They are better in a warm bed and with hot applications.

SILICA

This remedy is useful in several first aid conditions, such as colds, sore throats, hay fever, splinters, and thorns lodged under the skin. It works to alleviate constipation, migraine, chronic headaches, and sinus trouble. It is suited for people who have problems facing up to their problems and prefer not to take responsibility for themselves. They feel worse being cold, uncovered, in cold weather, and approaching winter. They are better when wrapped up, lying down, and in the summer.

SPONGIA

This remedy is used for coughs and croup. It is particularly good for children who continue to cough after the flu or a bad cold. There can be anxiety, difficulty breathing, and weakness after the slightest exertion. They are worse when ascending, in wind, after midnight, and are better descending and lying with head low. Children will hang their head over the bed to stop the coughing.

SULPHUR

This remedy has been used since ancient times to treat skin conditions: itching skin, rashes, acne, burning and itching hemorrhoids. It is useful for treating burning pains, tinnitus, diarrhea, and a lack of energy. It is excellent for colds that go directly into the lungs. It is suited to people who are deep thinkers and have a nervous yet independent nature. The person is worse in damp, cold weather and at the sea. They are better in warmth and fresh air.

SYMPHYTUM

This is used specifically to speed up the knitting of bones.

TARANTULA CUBENSIS

This is an effective remedy for boils, abscesses, or swelling where the tissue becomes blue and there are strong burning sensations. The patient is worse at night and is better when smoking.

TOBACCUM

This is used for the treatment of sea and motion sickness.

BACH FLOWER REMEDIES

These are distilled from flowers. *Rescue Remedy,* used most prevalently in first aid, is distilled from *Clematis,* which focuses on dizziness or loss of consciousness; *Cherry Plum,* which addresses loss of physical/mental control; *Impatiens,* which helps with emotional tension and pain; *Rock Rose,* which helps with panic and anxiety; and *Star of Bethlehem,* which works with physical trauma and loss and grief. *Rescue Remedy* is highly effective and works instantly in all sorts of physical, emotional, or upsetting circumstances. It can be applied to a wound or taken for any stress problems that shock the body or mind. It is useful at funerals, births, or any intense moment when a person is not themselves. *Rescue Remedy* is considered as important as *Arnica* for any first aid emergency.

COLOR REMEDIES

These have their own specific physical and emotional therapeutics.

Red is used for pain and problems with joints and ligaments of the feet, ankles, knees, and hips. It is useful for rectal problems, childbirth, postpartum care, varicose veins, hemorrhoids, and circulatory and autoimmune deficiency diseases. *Red* is useful wherever there is disharmony with the vital energy because of not being a part of a place, family, or community. It is useful for weakened life links, suicidal feelings, chronic and deep depression, and for acute and prolonged grief.

Orange is useful for sexual problems for both sexes, period pains, lower backache, allergies, constipation and sluggish bowels, anorexia and eating disorders, low vitality during post-operative care, autoimmune deficiency, poverty consciousness, joylessness, depressive weaknesses, and mobility difficulty.

Yellow is useful for liver, gallbladder, stomach, and pancreas problems, absorption problems, such as ciliac disease, and for osteoporosis, right eye problems, vision loss, decongestion of colds, and pulmonary problems. It is a good general detoxifier, ego booster for lack of confidence, for fear, agitation, and angry states. It increases intelligence, inner strength, and independence.

Green is used as a general diuretic for edematous conditions, especially pulmonary and cardiac conditions, as a cardiac regulator and toner, detoxifier, calmative, and tranquilizer. It helps promote a peaceful nature and passive spirit that is always seeking neutrality and avoiding change, and helps those gentle spirits who get weakened easily by life.

Turquoise works on the throat and mouth. It is good for catarrhal conditions, sore throats, and tired voices. It stimulates the thyroid and parathyroid glands, and is good for substance abuse cases where the patient wants to stop smoking, doing drugs, or over- or undereating. It is good for creative expression, lack of will power, integrity issues such as malicious gossiping, lying, and for shy communicators—those who need to speak up for themselves and express their feelings.

Indigo is good for tuning the senses, and acts as a calmative and anti-insomniac remedy. It is good for sinus problems, fevers, congestion of the head, eyestrain, and acts as a general anti-inflammatory. It works to instill wisdom, discernment, detachment, emotional distance, sensory acuity, imagination, intuition, clarity of mind, and to relieve timidity.

Violet is an antiseptic good for helping wounds heal, for tired nerves, and for improving the eyesight. It is a good anti-nausea remedy, for jaundice and liver conditions. It promotes peace, serenity, beauty, and spiritual awareness. It is good for excessive ego problems and chronic dull perceptions of life. It opens the spirit.

Pink is a good remedy for heart patients to ease fear and tension of heart disease. It is good for new mothers to help increase milk and attune them to motherhood. It opens the heart to sweetness, softness, and tenderness, and is good for difficult mother-daughter relationships, and for children who have been abandoned and abused.

Magenta is a good remedy for sexual, heart, and mind issues. It acts as a tonic for the lower centers and is good for the higher levels of thinking. It is an excellent remedy for creative and original people. It helps open one to change.

Spectrum is an overall tonic for burnout, autoimmune deficiency diseases, and post-viral or trauma conditions. It is used for substance abuse, overwork, and emotional difficulties which drain the vitality.

Cases

There are many stories about the effectiveness of homeopathic remedies, particularly in first aid. Nearly everyone familiar with homeopathy has an *Arnica* story. This remedy has been used by so many people in different situations that it is difficult to choose the best stories. I used *Arnica* for the first time when I slammed my fingers in a car door. I thought I would faint from the pain and feared losing a nail. I was given *Arnica* repeatedly over the next few hours and all the pain disappeared. This was followed by the discoloration disappearing. Finally, after a few hours, there was no pain or any sign that there had been an injury. I marveled at this remedy's capacity to heal. Another time I cut the soft skin between my thumb and first finger with the lid of a cat food can. The blood was spurting everywhere. I took *Arnica* and the bleeding stopped instantly, though the pain was severe. Another dose of *Arnica* and all the pain was gone. All this transpired within five minutes. Again, I can only marvel at its speed and efficiency.

I remember the case of a young father hit in the eye with a baseball. This man had no interest in homeopathy. His wife phoned for my advice. He was given *Arnica* every ten minutes until the pain began to disappear, and then he took it every hour until the swelling disappeared. After that he was to take it every two hours. The next morning he called personally to thank me and to make an appointment for a consultation. He was very impressed with the remedy. He said he was worried he would lose his eye, and twenty-four hours later he was wondering what all the fuss was about. The swelling had completely gone and he was left with a slightly red, but not seriously discolored eye.

A man was horseback riding with a homeopath friend. He fell off his horse and broke his arm. The homeopath had only two remedies: *Rescue Remedy* and *Arnica*. He administered both of these and took his companion to the hospital, where the break was set. The patient said that after these remedies he suffered no pain and was content to get back on his horse, ride to the car, and go to the hospital without feeling ill or panicky.

Arnica is used by the British Royal Air Force when the men are out on missions. I heard a medic from the Army talk about how he had used *Arnica* during the bombing of the Royal Barracks in Northern Ireland. He said that after the bomb exploded the calamity was intense and it was difficult to know who was alive or dead. He took an *Arnica* tablet and put it on the tongue of every person he could see. He says the fatalities were very low, to everyone's surprise. He attributes this to *Arnica*'s ability to alleviate shock. The young medic began to study homeopathy in London because he felt that it was worth the time and money.

A family on holiday was traveling by car when they were hit head-on. The mother was a homeopath and carried a first aid kit. She administered both *Arnica* and *Aconite* to her children (*Arnica* for shock with no fear, *Aconite* for shock with fear), and used

Rescue Remedy as well. She said the car was a total loss, but the family was fine. By the time the ambulance had arrived at the scene, the family had recovered from cuts, bruises, and shock.

A friend reported recently that *Merc. Sol* had completely stopped his toothache.

A secretary at a busy office who was prone to headaches found relief from her persistent headache with *Bryonia*. Many people who suffer headaches report how one dose of *Bryonia* helped alleviate all pain. They are never without it in their kits.

Another friend reported she had a tooth pulled, took *Arnica* the moment she left the dentist's office, and then in twelve to twenty minutes thereafter. After three repeated doses, she needed no aspirin. Vicodin had been prescribed because the dentist feared the pain would be dreadful.

A young mother of a toddler swears that no mother should be without *Chamomilla* for a teething child. She said that her irritable child calmed down after a single dose one evening when a new tooth was trying to come through.

She also later reported that *Belladonna* stopped a fever from developing in the same child when he had come home from child care with a fever and symptoms of cold and flu. She gave the child hot milk and one dose of *Belladonna* before putting him to bed. He slept all night and awoke in the morning feeling fine.

There are many testimonies to the wonders of *Arsen. Alb* for stopping an asthma attack in the middle of the night. It is also used for cases of restlessness when the patient can't settle into sleep. It is a remedy, like most of the first aid remedies, that is capable of covering many symptoms. It has a secure place in the treatment of the flu as well as treating those times when you feel drained of energy.

When you treat yourself with these remedies you will become familiar with how they work. You will have your own amazing stories to tell about how the remedies worked for you. With homeopathy you can feel secure about the quality and effectiveness of these remedies. They are meant to assist you and your family to achieve high levels of health and stability.

The less you are dependent upon doctors and drugs to "fix" your ailments, the more you can envision having good health and dealing with first aid situations quickly and effectively before they turn into a chronic condition. A good stock of first aid remedies can make the difference in getting over something quickly or prolonging the illness.

If a homeopathic remedy does not relieve symptoms, consult your physician.

Resources

A FIRST AID KIT

The following remedies can make a very basic first aid kit
(6x potency):

Aconite	Carbo Veg
Arnica	Ignatia
Arsen. Alb	Nux Vom
Belladonna	Rhus Tox
Bryonia	Ruta Grav

HOMEOPATHIC REMEDY SOURCES

These are some of the sources for obtaining remedies. Your
health food store and whole food grocery store stock remedies.
If you wish further information contact the following organizations.

Pharmacies

Boiron
6 Campus Blvd.
Newtown Square, PA 19073
1-800-258-8823

Dolisos America
3014 Rigel Ave.
Las Vegas, NV 89102
1-800-365-4767

Standard Homeopathic Company
154 W. 131st Street
Los Angeles, CA 90061
1-800-624-9659

For more information about where to find a registered homeopath, or homeopathic seminars and conferences contact: The National Center for Homeopathy (1-703-548-7790).

About the Author

Ambika Wauters is a registered classical homeopath, trained in the UK. She graduated with a dip. Hom. BD from the School of Homeopathic Medicine, Darlington, N. Yorks. She maintained a private clinic for ten years in Britain, and lectured at the Cranfield School of Business Management, Cranfield University, Bedforshire, UK, to businesspeople on the benefits of homeopathy. She has worked for international and national business organizations, including Visa International, as a consultant in homeopathy. She has done innovative work in developing homeopathic color remedies. Her books include:

Healing with the Energy of the Chakras
Chakras and Their Archetypes
Homeopathic Color Remedies
Lifechanges
Inner Radiance, Outer Beauty

These books are published by The Crossing Press. Her other books include: *The Angel Oracle*, published by St. Martin's Press, *The Chakra Oracle*, published by Conari Press, and *The Principles of Color Healing*, Harper-Collins. Ambika offers seminars in healing and life change.

She is director of an online course on Spiritual Homeopathy and has developed a line of homeopathic color remedies that work on the human energy system to restore balance and bring harmony where it is lacking. Homeopathic Color Remedies can be purchased directly from the author. A set of ten remedies come in 6x, 12c, and 30c potency and cost $50 plus $3 for postage.

She now has a homeopathic consulting practice in Boulder, Colorado.

If you wish further information regarding her workshops on the human energy system and the training she offers, as well as information concerning Spiritual Homeopathy or Lifechanges, contact her at:

P.O. Box 1371

Boulder, Colorado 80306-1371

Or visit her website at: ambikawauters.com

BOOKS BY THE CROSSING PRESS

OTHER BOOKS BY THE CROSSING PRESS

Balance Hormones Naturally
By Kate Neil and Patrick Holford

Nutrition experts Kate Neil and Patrick Holford show you how to treat: premenstrual tension and depression, irregular and heavy periods, infertility, weight gain and bloating, menopause problems, breast lumps and cancer, ovarian cysts and fibroids, and other women's problems by using one simple medicine-food. In this breakthrough book, you will get the information you need to overcome the health issues that all women face today.

$12.95 • Paper • ISBN 1-58091-041-6

Color and Crystals: A Journey Through the Chakras
By Joy Gardner-Gordon

Information about color, crystals, tones, personality types, and Tarot archetypes that correspond to each chakra. Fully illustrated, indexed and well-organized.

$14.95 • Paper • ISBN 0-89594-258-5

The Essence of Bach Flowers: Traditional and Transpersonal Use and Practice
By Rachelle Hasnas

The Essence of Bach Flowers brings new understanding to what healing really is about. Hasna's combining of the traditional use of Bach's flower essences with metaphysical practice allows us to take responsibility for our health in a new holistic way.

$16.95 • Paper •ISBN 0-89594-969-5

Essential Reiki: A Complete Guide to an Ancient Healing Art
By Diane Stein

This bestseller includes the history of Reiki, hand positions, giving treatments, and the initiations. While no book can replace directly received attunements, Essential Reiki provides everything else that the practitioner and teacher of this system needs, including all three degrees of Reiki, most of it in print for the first time.

$18.95 • Paper • ISBN 0-89594-736-6

BOOKS BY THE CROSSING PRESS

Healing with Color Zone Therapy

By Joseph Corvo and Lilian Verner-Bonds

Corvo and Verner-Bonds introduce a form of therapy that treats the whole person: the physical, the emotional, and the spiritual. The safe, step-by-step techniques of Color Zone Therapy are followed by an A-Z list of charts for more than one hundred common ailments.

$14.95 • Paper • ISBN 0-89594-925-3

Healing with Flower and Gemstone Essences

By Diane Stein

Instructions for choosing and using flowers and gems are combined with descriptions of their effect on emotional balance. Includes instructions for making flower essences and for matching essences to hara line chakras for maximum benefit.

$14.95 • Paper • ISBN 0-89594-856-7

The Healing Energy of Your Hands

By Michael Bradford

Bradford offers techniques so simple that anyone can work with healing energy quickly and easily.

$12.95 • Paper • ISBN 0-89594-781-1

Healing Yourself Naturally

By Judy Jacka

From acne to warts, this book gives a clear explanation of the natural way to deal with illness and disease. Judy Jacka's book rests on the holistic view that the body can balance itself, the aim of naturopathy being to help the body do exactly that. Each disorder is listed alphabetically with a description of symptoms, causes, treatments, and case histories.

$18.95 • Paper • ISBN 0-89594-954-7

The Herbal Menopause Book: Herbs, Nutrition, and Other Natural Therapies

By Amanda McQuade Crawford

This comprehensive volume provides dozens of specific herbal remedies and other natural therapies for women facing the health issues that arise in pre-menopause, menopause, and post menopause.

$16.95 • Paper • ISBN 0-89594-799-4

Books by The Crossing Press

The Information Sourcebook of Herbal Medicine
By David Hoffman, B.Sc., M.N.I.M.H.

A comprehensive guide to information on western herbal medicine, offering a bibliography of herbalism and herbal pharmacology, a glossary of herbal and medical terms, computer databases for the herbalist, and Medline citations for commonly used medicinal herbs.

$40.00 • Hardcover • ISBN 0-89594-671-8

The Natural Remedy Book for Women
By Diane Stein

This bestselling, self-help guide to holistic health care includes information on ten different natural healing methods. Remedies from all ten methods are given for fifty common health problems.

$16.95 • Paper • ISBN 0-89594-525-8

The Optimum Nutrition Bible
By Patrick Holford

Optimum nutrition is a revolution in health care. It means giving yourself the best possible intake of nutrients to allow your body to be as healthy as possible. *The Optimum Nutrition Bible* shows you precisely how to achieve this, and gives a step-by-step plan to create your own personal supplement program. The results will speak for themselves.

$16.95 • Paper • ISBN 1-58091-015-7

Pocket Guide to Bach Flower Essences
By Rachelle Hasnas

Bach flower essences provide a remarkable form of energetic healing for yourself, your family and pets. You can learn how to select appropriate flower essences with confidence and use them to bring your body, mind and spirit into harmony.

$6.95 • Paper • ISBN 0-89594-865-6

Pocket Guide to Chakras
By Joy Gardner-Gordon

This book will answer your questions about chakra, including explaining what they are, where they are, how they function and what causes the chakras to open and close.

$6.95 • Paper • ISBN 0-89594-949-0

BOOKS BY THE CROSSING PRESS

OTHER BOOKS BY AMBIKA WAUTERS

Chakras and Their Archetypes: Uniting Energy Awareness and Spiritual Growth

By Ambika Wauters

Linking classic archetypes to the seven chakras in the human energy system can reveal unconscious ways of behaving. Wauters helps us understand where our energy is blocked, which attitudes or emotional issues are responsible, and how to then transcend our limitations.

$16.95 • Paper • ISBN 0-89594-891-5

Healing with the Energy of the Chakras

By Ambika Wauters

Chakras are swirling wheels of light and color—vortices through which energy must pass in order to nourish and maintain physical, emotional, mental and spiritual life. Wauters presents a self-help program intended to give you guidelines and a framework within which to explore and understand more about how your energetic system responds to thoughts and expression.

$14.95 • Paper • ISBN 0-89594-906-7

Homeopathic Color Remedies

By Ambika Wauters

Color has been known to have a strong influence on people and treatment with colored light has been used in naturopathic circles for several decades. Wauters' homeopathic color remedies serve as medicine for our energy body, increasing the energetic flow physically, emotionally, and mentally.

$12.95 • Paper • ISBN 0-89594-997-0

LifeChanges with the Energy of the Chakras

By Ambika Wauters

When we face up to the reality of change, we learn to accept its challenges with grace and renewed grit. We can alter our old movies-our old patterns-and gain insights into our nature. We then can be released from the past and find new, healthy options for our lives.

$14.95 • Paper • ISBN 1-58091-020-3

To receive a current catalog from The Crossing Press
please call toll-free, 800-777-1048.
Visit our Web site: **www.crossingpress.com**